# THE
# **COSMETIC SURGERY**
# COMPANION

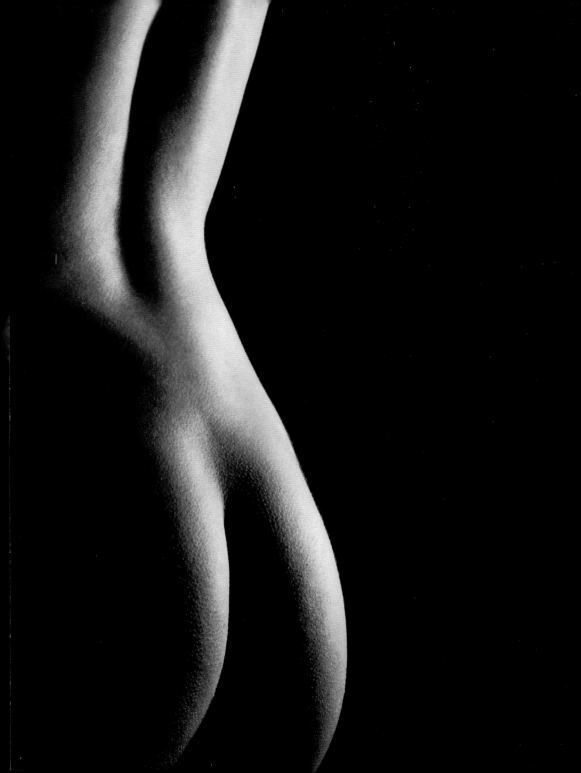

# THE
# **COSMETIC SURGERY**
# COMPANION

**Antonia Mariconda**

FIREFLY BOOKS

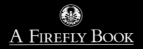

## A FIREFLY BOOK

Published by Firefly Books Ltd. 2010
Copyright © 2010 Quintet Publishing

First printing, 2010

Publisher Cataloging-in-Publication Data
(U.S.)

Mariconda, Antonia.

The cosmetic surgery companion : a
consumer's guide to the latest surgical
techniques to improve your body from head
to toe / Antonia Mariconda.

[256] p. :  col. photos. ;  cm.

Includes index.

Summary: An essential resource for those in
search of the body beautiful, tackling every
question, *The Cosmetic Surgery Companion*
describes the surgical options available for
improving each body zone, as well as
explaining a range of alternative solutions
so that the reader can make an informed
choice about what's right for them.

ISBN-13: 978-1-55407-524-9

ISBN-10: 1-55407-524-6

1. Surgery, Plastic – Popular works.  I. Title.
617.95 dc22   RD119.M375   2010

Library and Archives Canada Cataloging in
Publication

Mariconda, Antonia

The cosmetic surgery companion : a
consumer's guide to the latest surgical
techniques to improve your body from head
to toe / Antonia Mariconda.

Includes index.

ISBN-13: 978-1-55407-524-9

ISBN-10: 1-55407-524-6

1. Surgery, Plastic--Popular works.  I. Title.
RD119.M37 2010          617.9'52
C2010-901657-2

Published in the United States by
Firefly Books (U.S.) Inc.
P.O. Box 1338, Ellicott Station
Buffalo, New York 14205

Published in Canada by
Firefly Books Ltd.
66 Leek Crescent
Richmond Hill, Ontario L4B 1H1

| | |
|---|---|
| Project editor | Liz Dalby |
| Designer | Bonnie Bryan |
| Illustrator | Bernard Chau |
| Art director | Michael Charles |
| Managing editor | Donna Gregory |
| Publisher | James Tavendale |

Printed in China

# Contents

# FOREWORDS

*The Cosmetic Surgery Companion*, by Antonia Mariconda, is a very well thought out overview of cosmetic surgery. It responsibly identifies clients likely to benefit from such procedures and has an emphasis on informed consent and patient safety. Choosing a good, local cosmetic surgeon is often better than traveling great distances to see a surgeon with a high media profile but with the same surgical ability. Complications may occur even with the "best" surgeons and swift, accessible aftercare is vital. The text is clear and concise and well set out to keep the reader's attention.

The photographs are a fair reflection of the average expected outcomes from surgery and do not glamorize the procedures. There has been a good deal of research in compiling the facts in this companion and, generally, they represent "state-of-the-art" knowledge. The emphasis is to encourage the right patient to proceed to the right surgery, under the right surgeon, in the right facility. Patient expectations must be realistic and surgeons must always think "Patient Safety First."

**Professor James D. Frame FRCS FRCS(Plast)**
**Consultant Plastic and Reconstructive Surgeon**
**Professor of Aesthetic Plastic Surgery,**
**Anglia Ruskin University, UK**

We live in a health-conscious society and there is a strong interest in looking as good as you feel; we're more aware than ever that making a good impression on others benefits us both socially and economically. In addition to diet and exercise, cosmetic procedures are becoming part of the whole healthcare philosophy. We are living longer, staying fitter, and leading more active lives. In simple terms, today, age does not really matter any more.

The increase in reality TV programs such as *Extreme Makeover* and *The Swan* has fueled the growing interest in and demand for cosmetic treatments, and magazines and newspapers are all too keen to display the latest nipped and tucked celebrities. Even upmarket publications such as Vogue run regular features on "what's hot" in the world of cosmetic enhancement, and Googling "cosmetic surgery" generates more than 7 million hits. Cosmetic enhancement is firmly entrenched in our culture. When it comes to cosmetic surgery I believe that information should be presented to the consumer in an honest, detailed, and thorough way. A cosmetic surgery patient who has conducted comprehensive research will not only be more likely to have realistic expectations, but is also likely to be happier with the outcome.

Cosmetic surgery procedures once thought to be "only for the rich and famous" are now commonly affordable and undertaken by men and women with average incomes who feel that they are investing in themselves.

While any elective surgical procedure carries some risk, the technological and procedural advances of recent years have translated into faster patient recovery, lower morbidity and mortality, and more natural-seeming results. Our fast-paced, competitive society has created a demand for nonsurgical procedures that have little or no downtime, allowing many people who would not have considered surgery in the past to be more open to having aesthetic enhancement.

The decision to have cosmetic surgery ultimately lies with you, and therefore the responsibility is yours alone. Making any alteration to your appearance should be a decision taken with great care, following careful consideration and research. Take your time when searching for a surgeon and make sure your expectations are realistic. We're all happier and more confident about life when we know we're fulfilling our own potential, and wanting a more appealing appearance in today's society is nothing new. Enjoy the journey of discovery, and good luck...

**Antonia Mariconda**

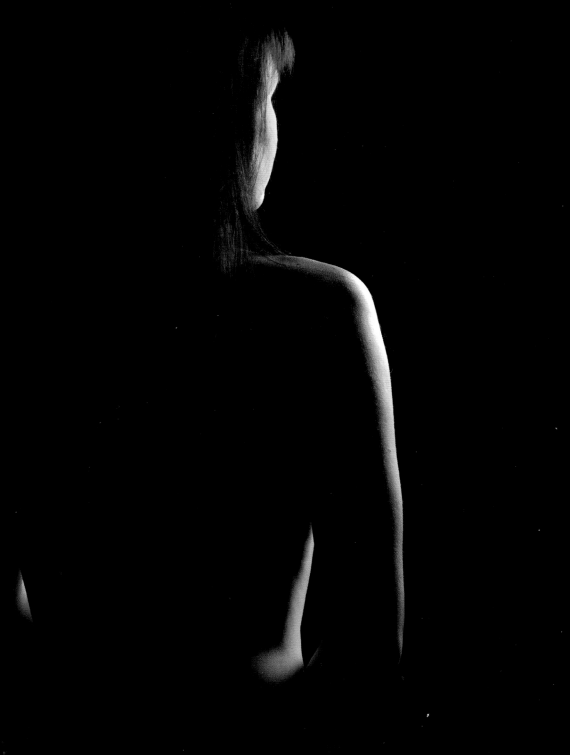

# CHAPTER ONE
# ABOUT COSMETIC SURGERY

# ABOUT COSMETIC SURGERY
*An overview*

**Cosmetic surgery is a constantly developing field of medicine dedicated to improving and rejuvenating the face and body. Unlike reconstructive surgery, which is concerned with the correction of defects caused by illness, accidents, or from birth, cosmetic surgery is largely about aesthetic enhancement.**

Some say, falsely, that such enhancements are "pure vanity." In fact, cosmetic surgery has incalculable value for patients who are made deeply unhappy by their looks: those who have, for example, been teased from childhood for an oddly shaped nose or sticking-out ears. Or those who may avoid ordinary social and sexual contact because they believe their acne scars or body flaws, such as asymmetric breasts, make them unacceptable to others.

Not least, in this competitive world, patients of both sexes seek surgery to look younger and avoid being considered "too old" for their work. Ageism may be frowned upon or legislated against, but it is still a very real threat to older employees.

And, of course, many patients simply want to improve the freshness and smoothness of their skin, the plumpness of their lips, and gain a general "uplift" of a face and body that has been eroded over the years.

## GAINING POPULARITY

Up until fairly recently, such surgery was largely viewed as an eccentric luxury and carried a stigma to the extent that people often went to great lengths to conceal their surgical self-improvement efforts. Today, however, thanks to the social acceptance of cosmetic surgery, it is not uncommon to overhear a cosmetic surgery patient telling anyone who will listen about her brand new breasts, or new improved nose.

Much of the ever-growing popularity of cosmetic surgery is down to the excellence of modern techniques and equipment, and to the high standards of the surgeons and other professional practitioners.

In the U.S., surgeons must be certified by the American Board of Plastic Surgery (ABPS), and they must have met stringent requirements. These include a good degree from an accredited medical school, the completion of at least 3 years of general surgery, 2 to 3 years of supervised plastic surgery residency, and 2 years of professional practice.

According to the ABPS website: "The plastic surgeon uses cosmetic surgical principles both to improve overall appearance and to optimize the outcome of reconstructive procedures. Anatomy, physiology, pathology, and other basic sciences are fundamental to the specialty."

## A LITTLE BACKGROUND

The first U.S. medical text about cosmetic procedures was written just over 100 years ago, when Dr. Charles Miller wrote about "The Correction of Feature Imperfections" in 1907. At that time, almost every aspect of cosmetic surgery was viewed with suspicion by the general public, and surgeons were accused of being "quacks."

But, as the years went by and techniques and procedures developed, the importance of this branch of medicine became evident.

Today, according to CBS News, nearly 11 million cosmetic procedures were performed in the U.S. alone, in 2006—an increase of 50 percent since 2000. A year later, in 2007, nearly 12 million procedures were carried out.

## POPULAR PROCEDURES

Procedures that are particularly popular in the U.S. are liposuction, breast augmentation (mammoplasty), eyelid surgery (blepharoplasty), facelift (rhytidectomy), nose reshaping (rhinoplasty), and tummy tuck (abdominoplasty).

The online Encyclopedia of Surgery says that procedures that improve the complexion are also in the "top ten"; this is largely due to advances in laser treatments and chemical peels. Skin disfigured by scars and pitting, or by sun damage, can be smoothed, freshened, and resurfaced.

## NEW TECHNIQUES

As well as the best-known cosmetic surgery applications, medical and scientific

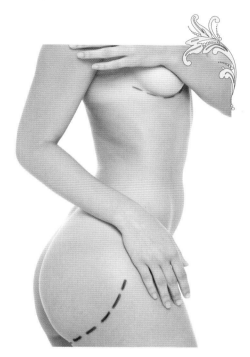

**Cosmetic surgery of the buttocks is increasing in popularity.**

advances mean that new techniques are being developed all the time. A buttock augmentation—often informally known as a "butt implant"—uses silicone or the patient's own fat to lift and improve the shape of the bottom. Arms and necks can be firmed and lifted, and there is even a dramatic procedure that involves lifting the torso to eliminate sagging. Fillers of collagen and other substances can be used to plump up the lips, while cheeks and the chin can be given more definition with carefully molded implants. And another interesting advance is that an increasing number of men are opting for facelifts, tummy tucks, man-breast reduction, and other procedures.

# HISTORY

There are two major branches of aesthetic surgery—cosmetic surgery and reconstructive surgery. The first has only come to the fore in recent decades, though its development has been quite extraordinarily swift and sure. Reconstructive surgery, by contrast, stretches back thousands of years and developed over centuries through trial and error. The history books record that the first reconstructive surgery procedures were performed in ancient Roman times.

One ancient Roman report told how a patient had repairs to his earlobes, which had grown excessively long after years of bearing heavy earrings. The lobes were trimmed and the patient must have decided "Never again!" as he asked for the holes in the lobes to be sewn up. Another, particularly expensive, treatment was one that was often undergone by freed slaves, who were only too glad to pay for the removal of the branding marks inflicted by their former owners.

There is also evidence that Indian physicians were skilled in the techniques of facial enhancement hundreds of years BCE. This also involved largely reconstructive work using skin grafts to repair damaged noses, ears, and lips.

However, it wasn't until the fifteenth century that a German physician named Heinrich von Pfolspeundt carried out the first European facial surgery—a rhinoplasty procedure to build a new nose for a patient. And in Italy in the same century, similar rebuilding and repairing techniques were being developed and refined.

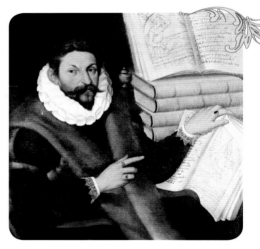

**Above: Gaspare Tagliacozzi.**
**Right: An illustration of an early rhinoplasty (nose surgery) procedure.**

Gasparo Tagliacozzi (1545–1599) wrote an important text on reconstructive surgery, which described how damaged facial features could be repaired or replaced using skin grafts. However, he incurred the wrath

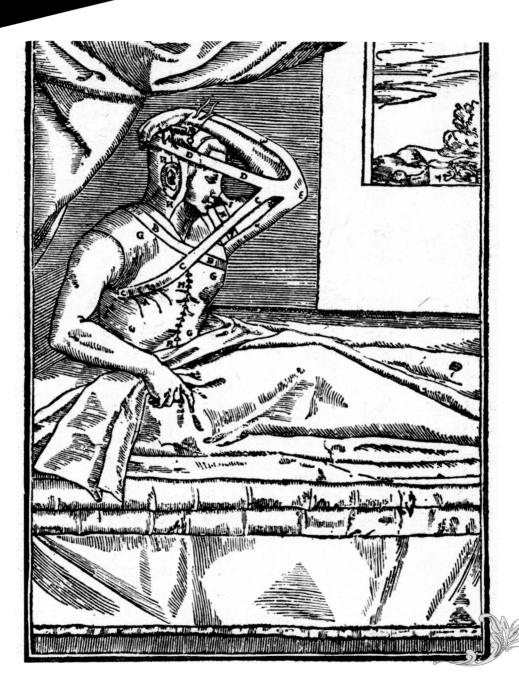

of the Church authorities, who believed such surgery was against the will of God. He was excommunicated after death, and his body removed from its grave in consecrated ground.

Sadly, like all medical procedures of the time, cosmetic surgery was a risky business. There was little or no knowledge of hygiene or the causes of infection, and there was of course no anesthetic.

## MODERN COSMETIC SURGERY

The first American plastic surgeon, John Mettauer, performed the world's first cleft palate operation in 1827. His was a huge step forward in the field of facial surgery—and Dr. Mettauer's work was especially impressive as he had designed the instruments he used himself.

Other U.S. pioneers were John Roe who, in around 1891, reduced a young woman's nose hump, and George Monks, who in the previous decade had worked on bone-grafting techniques to improve sunken noses.

However, the great leap forward in reconstructive surgery came during World War I; one of the founders of modern techniques, American Vilray Blair, treated soldiers there with complex facial injuries. He afterward wrote a paper, "Reconstructive Surgery of the Face," and this set the standard for craniofacial reconstruction for years to come. Vilray

Blair went on to teach many other surgeons who became famed for their expertise in reconstructive surgery.

Today such surgery is performed for many reasons, including repairing congenital abnormalities and improving limb function, largely through skin grafts, for burns patients. Cleft palate surgery and breast reconstruction after mastectomy are also common procedures.

Aesthetic cosmetic surgery was rarely performed until the early years of the last century. It was simply too dangerous to attempt non-vital surgery when the risks of any type of surgery were so great. However, the experiences of surgeons working with World War I soldiers brought a new awareness of how facial damage can impact dreadfully on self-esteem. Soldiers whose faces were wrecked in the battleground were profoundly affected, their confidence lost. This led to a new respect for purely aesthetic procedures.

Around the same time, the importance of hygiene was fully recognized, and antiseptics and antibiotics were working their magic. Meanwhile, cosmetic surgery pioneers were developing their skills and techniques. As the years went by, procedures became ever more sophisticated, safe, and effective.

The earliest purely cosmetic operations included rhinoplasty and breast augmentation. Both saline and silicone

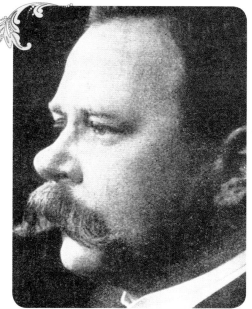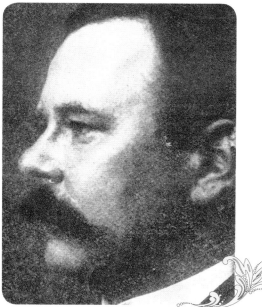

**Above: Examples of cosmetic surgery carried out in Paris in 1907. The procedure was carried out under a local anesthetic, typically cocaine.**

breast implants were introduced in the 1960s, and liposuction followed some 20 years later. Also, from the mid-twentieth century, surgeons were able to help their patients enhance their appearance through facelifts, tummy tucks, and eye-bag removal.

Procedures have developed greatly over the years. Silicone breast implants, for example, are much safer today, because they are usually made of high-cohesive gel. This is thicker than other types of silicone and reduces the chance of leakage. Fluid injections for liposuction have had a double advantage: there is no longer the need for a general anesthetic, yet patients will usually have fat cells more efficiently removed.

Indeed, liposuction, together with lip enhancement, has been one of the most popular cosmetic procedures in recent years. Techniques to improve the complexion are also sought after, as chemical peels and lasers become ever more fine-tuned, safe, and effective. Advances in cosmetic surgery mean that every year, there are quicker and more sophisticated ways to treat patients.

# ADVANCES AND DEVELOPMENTS IN COSMETIC SURGERY

**Cosmetic surgery is one of the fastest-developing fields in medicine. Techniques, skills, and the "tools of the trade" are constantly being refined and improved. It is widely acknowledged that no branch of medical science has made such dramatic advancements in such a relatively short space of time.**

Recent advances range from the breathtakingly complex—such as whole-face transplantation—to subtle, less invasive liposuction procedures. Hugely significant for the future is the use of stem cells to grow new tissue that exactly matches your existing body, while facelifts are entering a new phase through the use of endoscopes.

Detailed information on the first U.S. facial transplantation was presented in the January 2010 issue of the journal *Plastic and Reconstructive Surgery*. Following five years of research and development, the transplant was carried out in Cleveland in December 2008, and appears to have been a complete success.

The other especially interesting cosmetic surgery development concerns the use of the patient's own stem cells. The website plasticsurgery.about.com offers a "short version" of how stem cell augmentation works: "A surgeon performs liposuction on an area of the body and the suctioned fat is divided in half. One half has its stem cells extracted and purified. The stem cells are then added and mixed into the other half of the fat, which is then introduced into the new site where more fullness is desired.

"The extra stem cells serve two purposes: to increase the amount of transplanted fat that survives and thrives, and to encourage growth of more fat cells in the transplant area; the end result is that you can actually grow your own bigger breasts. Your own fat and stem cells are used and there is no need for the introduction of any foreign of artificial materials into your body. Bonus—you get a flatter tummy or thinner thighs, as the case may be, as a result of the liposuction portion of the procedure."

At present, the procedure is still in the experimental stage. But the endoscope facial rejuvenation technique is already transforming this branch of facial surgery.

As for liposuction developments, the "tumescent technique" means a surgeon expands the fat and tissues with local anesthesia, adrenaline, and salt water. This reduces blood loss and increases the amount of fat that can be removed, without the need for a general anesthetic.

More advances are explained at medicalnewstoday.com. A U.S. rhinoplasty specialist has, it says, revolutionized rhinoplasty by eliminating traditional packing. Many potential rhinoplasty patients

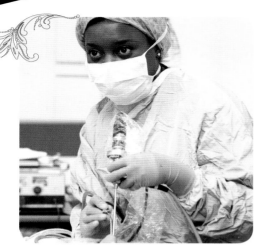

**The field of cosmetic surgery is constantly improving, with frequent technical innovations.**

are so concerned about the pain associated with the post-operative removal of nasal packing that they postpone or even avoid surgery. However, the new technique means that plant-based biopolymer materials with super-absorbent qualities can eliminate the need for painful packing removal.

Recent trends in cosmetic surgery involve the shift of emphasis from complex surgical procedures to minimally invasive techniques—and prospects for the coming decades seem even better. Procedures are increasingly becoming quicker, requiring less downtime for recovery. Scarring is going to be less and expenses are also coming down significantly, attracting a larger segment of society.

Research is moving toward the most advanced kind of cosmetic engineering. For example, scientists have achieved

major breakthroughs in the area of tissue engineering that will make generation of live tissues possible in the lab, to be used to replace damaged skin and body parts.

Research is also being carried out to explore the possibilities of reproducing skin grafts, breast tissue, muscles, or nerves. Thus the future of cosmetic surgery seems to mostly depend on the advancements made in the area of tissue engineering.

In the years to come, techniques are predicted to develop at an ever faster rate. More advanced approaches are expected to replace the present techniques as demand for procedures with immediate effects and quicker healing times grows. Along with the advances in treatments, there are significant improvements in the surgeons' abilities to communicate with their patients. One tool for aiding such communication has been the new computer software that allows a physician to take digital photographs of a patient and modify their image on a computer screen. With this technique a surgeon can show a patient an image of a reasonable outcome of any given cosmetic procedure. The patient can also show the doctor what they like or dislike about the current features or about the potential outcome of a procedure.

Those working in the cosmetic surgery industry—researchers, technicians, scientists, laboratory specialists, and surgeons—are constantly examining all possible ways to improve the effectiveness and optimize the results of procedures. Not long ago, no one imagined such procedures as chin augmentation or buttock lifts, dermal fillers, or hair transplantation.

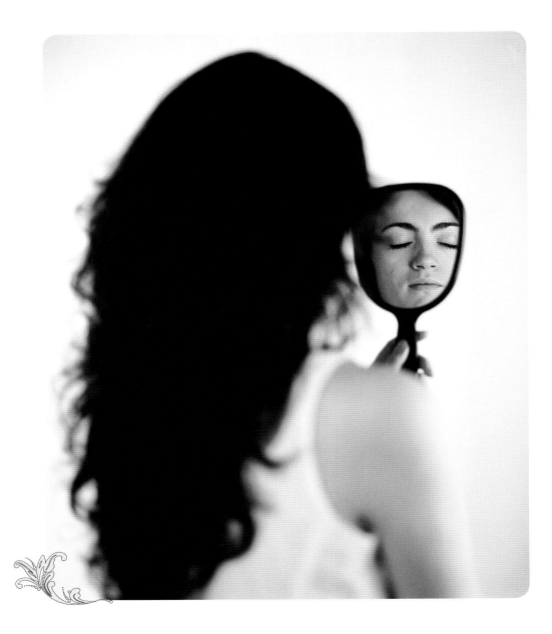

The decision to have cosmetic surgery should never be undertaken lightly. Cosmetic surgery can change your appearance in ways that you might consider desirable but it can also take a long time, be expensive, and—although quite rare—it has been known to result in appearance changes that you may not always find pleasing in the future. It is important that you do not feel pressured into having cosmetic surgery, nor is it wise to rush into making a choice without extensive research; it should be a decision you make only after a lot of careful thought and questioning.

If you have decided that cosmetic surgery is for you this is probably because you have identified something about yourself that you consider to be a flaw; however, consider this evaluation carefully. A "flaw" should be something that really bothers you; if it is something you can live with then think again about whether cosmetic surgery really is the solution. However, if it is something you think about on a daily basis, to the point that it is constantly on your mind, perhaps you are ready for an improvement. In the process of considering your motivations and objectives for having cosmetic surgery it is important that you know exactly what is of concern to you about the way you look and that you are able to describe this to the surgeon. It might be helpful to consider the questions that follow when making your evaluation.

## WHAT BOTHERS ME ABOUT MY FACE AND BODY?

There is no one better than yourself to make a detailed analysis of your face and body. Making a list of the things you do not like about yourself is the best way to see

clearly what concerns you about the way you look. You might find this a worthwhile exercise to carry out by yourself first; somewhere along the line you will have to explain your concerns to the cosmetic surgeon(s) you meet and consult with, and your final decision will hinge on these concerns and the surgeon's subsequent recommendations and advice. You may end up with a very short list, or a long one, but asking yourself what really bothers you will help you to establish your priorities.

## HOW MUCH DO I REALLY WANT TO CHANGE THE THINGS THAT BOTHER ME?

This is a question only you can answer, and will depend on the impact your image concerns have on your life. For example, if your concerns cause you deep psychological problems or severe embarrassment to the point that they limit your social enjoyment and daily life, then your motivations for wanting to change will be quite strong. If, however, you are someone with image concerns but you generally do not allow them to impact your daily life and social enjoyment, then ask yourself if cosmetic surgery is really something you want to do; consider that there might be alternative solutions to help you address your concerns.

Weigh up your motivations for wanting to change the issues that truly bother you about the way you look against the cost of cosmetic surgery, the possible risks and complications, and the recovery and healing times.

## HAVE I CONSIDERED ALL THE OPTIONS?

Cosmetic surgery is not the only option available to you. This is something that the cosmetic surgeons that you consult should point out to you, and you may also find that cosmetic surgeons will suggest alternative ways to address your concerns. Understanding all your options gives you a better chance of making a decision you are happy with. Don't be afraid to request a second consultation with a surgeon, to clarify any advice you have been given, and to research alternative solutions and treatments suggested to you before making that final decision.

## WHAT WILL MY FRIENDS AND FAMILY THINK OF ME FOR CHOOSING COSMETIC SURGERY?

It is not uncommon for friends and family members to be worried once you have informed them of your decision to have cosmetic surgery—after all, with your best interests at heart they are more likely to focus on the risks, complications, and your general safety more than any other factor such as the motivations behind your decision or the surgical result. It may not be easy for you to listen to the opinions and concerns your family and friends convey to you. The opinions of people close to you can weigh heavily upon you, especially at a time when you are trying to remain focused on the surgical outcome and positive in respect of the decision you have made. However, try to understand their concerns—after all, it is because they care about you. Talk about the information you have gathered and researched that helped you arrive at your decision and welcome their questions; talking openly and honestly may serve as a useful exercise to both parties in feeling reassured about the decision.

## CAN I KEEP MY COSMETIC SURGERY A SECRET?

As tempting as it is to want to keep your cosmetic surgery a secret, it might not be as easy as you think. You may want to consider being open about the procedures you are going to have simply to avoid the stress of having to hide away until all visible bruises and other signs of surgery have vanished. It may also be the most plausible explanation for the suddenly flat and tight tummy, the streamlined body contour, or the new nose. Bear in mind too that the

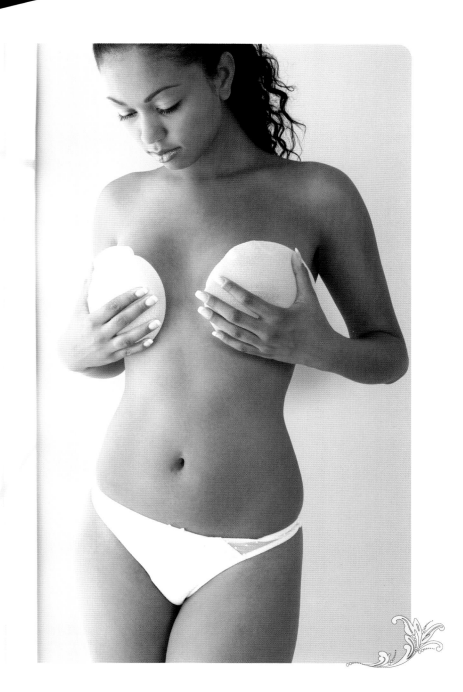

more cosmetic work you have done the harder it may be to keep secret.

If you do choose, for whatever reason, to keep your surgery quiet, then carefully plan your recovery. Consider a vacation after surgery—the relaxation of a holiday break and a tan will help you recover and give you a refreshed glow when you return to face friends and family. Do ensure that if you are recovering from surgery at home by yourself that you have plenty of help and assistance at hand; with some cosmetic surgery procedures strict recovery instructions must be followed for optimum recovery and personal safety.

## AM I PREPARED FOR THE FINANCIAL COST OF COSMETIC SURGERY?

If you have been considering cosmetic surgery for some time, you will have factored the cost into your decision. If you have saved the money for your procedure and you are willing to spend it to make yourself look and feel better then that is good; however, if you do not have the funds readily available for your chosen procedure(s) then you may want to consider several options for funding your surgery so you can move forward with your plans. Many cosmetic surgery clinics and surgeons now offer flexible finance options and plans whereby you can pay for your surgery on a monthly credit basis; alternatively many banks and building societies now offer loans for people considering cosmetic surgery.

It is not advisable to put yourself under financial stress if you do not have the means to pay for your surgery in the long run, as this could affect your credit rating and harm your financial status in the future. Having this worry, in addition to your recovery and healing, is not ideal. The best solution may be to plan, save, and wait until you are in a position where you can comfortably afford the surgical procedures without placing yourself under any unnecessary stress or liability.

## HOW WOULD I DEAL WITH ANY COMPLICATIONS?

All surgery, no matter what kind, carries the risk of complications. If you are unfortunate enough to be one of the patients who experience a rare serious complication as a result of your cosmetic surgery, you must be prepared to deal with it. It is essential that you accept that complications can happen. If you feel that you are not physically or emotionally equipped to deal with a possible complication, which could result in anything from delayed healing time, to additional surgery, or serious side effects—simply don't do it. It is impossible to predict what complications will occur following any type of surgery, as each individual patient responds to recovery and healing in a very unique and different way.

The most important precaution you can take is to find a reputable, qualified surgeon with a good team of staff whom you feel you can trust to take good care of you.

## HOW CAN I TAKE TIME OUT TO RECOVER?

The fast pace of modern life makes it hard to imagine taking the time out to recover from cosmetic surgery; responsibilities including families, relationships, work, and social commitments mean that in reality very few people have the time for recovery. But with careful planning you can create the recovery time you need. Your surgeon will give you an idea of the necessary recovery and healing time when you have your initial consultation.

With forward planning you can book time off work if you need to, or if you have a family you can schedule surgery around a time when you can draft in help from family or friends. If you follow your surgeon's recovery instructions carefully,

healing will be smoother; however, factor in the possibility of complications, and extra recovery time may be needed. Ask yourself if your employer or family would be able to accept that in the unlikely event that it happened.

## HOW WILL I FIND THE RIGHT SURGEON?

If you have decided, after careful evaluation, that cosmetic surgery is something you want to do, then perhaps the most important aspect of your experience is finding a reputable, qualified, and skilled surgeon. See pages 28–35 for much more about finding a surgeon.

You should see more than one surgeon and have more than one consultation with each surgeon you talk to. Also try to speak to friends and family and to people that have had cosmetic surgery and can relay their experiences to you. The Internet is also a valuable resource for those researching cosmetic surgery. Arming yourself with information and knowledge is key.

### SUMMARY

Be honest with yourself—making a realistic evaluation about the way you feel and look is the most important part of making such an important and life-changing decision; a decision over which you have control.

There are millions of people who have experienced the life-changing and positive effect that cosmetic

surgery can have on their lives, but such successful outcomes really do come from the right emotional and physiological foundation being firmly in place from the outset. If you are a physically and psychologically healthy adult, with the financial means to afford cosmetic surgery, then it may be the option for you.

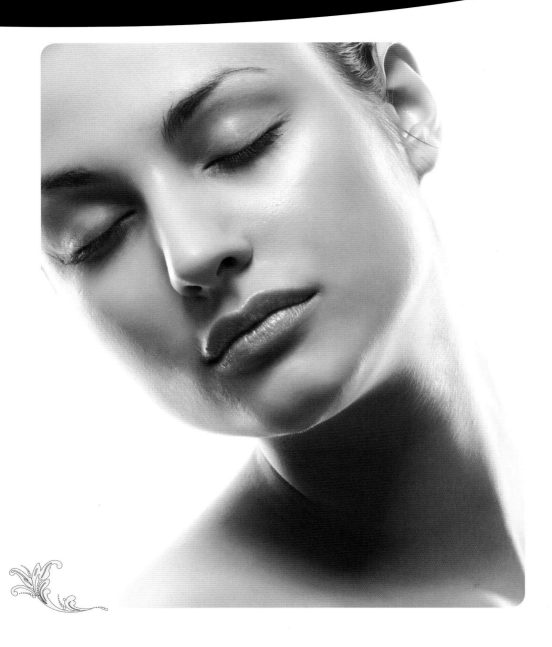

**To opt for surgery—or not to opt for surgery? That is, ultimately, the question. Just about anyone who has considered undergoing cosmetic procedures—whether noninvasive or surgical—has weighed up the risks against the rewards. In fact, reputable surgeons will turn away patients who haven't thought the issues through.**

For such treatments as laser or dermabrasion skin correction, the considerations are largely whether the soreness will be bearable, the recovery time acceptable, and the end result worth the effort. But for procedures that involve anesthetic and a scalpel, it is sensible to give serious thought to both the short- and long-term health implications.

For a start, what are the health risks? What is the success rate of this type of operation and what—in a worst-case scenario—could possibly go wrong? Do expectations match reality? Are your hopes for a smooth, flat tummy or a fresher, younger-looking face going to be realized?

Certified cosmetic surgeons are not only highly skilled but are also attuned to the needs, hopes, and fears of their patients. They should explain the procedures, describe the risks, offer reassurance, and give their honest assessment of the result of the operation. The surgery process only goes ahead when both physician and patient are in accord.

## GENERAL RISKS

Call it "reconstructive," "cosmetic," or "plastic"—it's still surgery. The worst outcomes are rare but risk is nonetheless a reality. While each type of surgery has its own risks specific to that particular procedure, certain risks are common to virtually all surgical procedures, including:

- Infection
- Excessive or unexpected bleeding
- Blood clots
- Tissue death
- Delayed healing
- Anesthesia risks including shock, respiratory failure, and cardiac arrest
- Pneumonia
- Need for secondary surgeries/ dissatisfaction with results
- Paralysis or less severe nerve damage
- As with all surgery, there is a risk of death

## PSYCHOLOGICALLY AT EASE?

**"How will you feel if your surgery makes you a subject of gossip in your social circle?"**

**"What if your partner exhibits signs of jealousy because of your improved looks?"**

**"Will you be perfectly comfortable with the increased attention you get with your newly enlarged breasts?"**

There are many emotional changes linked to cosmetic surgery. Choosing cosmetic surgery to improve a bodily or facial flaw is one thing; choosing it with an expectation of improving the rest of your life is another.

However, the good news is that a study by the American Society of Plastic Surgeons found that 75 percent of the respondents indicated that they chose surgery to gain an improved appearance and a more active lifestyle. Likewise, 70 percent cited emotional and physical rewards after surgery, with notable increases in happiness, renewed self-esteem, and more confidence. Equally impressive, 45 percent enjoyed the daily benefit of being more attractive.

This, of course, is why millions of people in the U.S. and elsewhere choose cosmetic surgery—to change the way they look, either facially or bodily, so that they can

enjoy a happier, more fulfilled life. It is acknowledged in the world of psychology that the best-looking people are generally the most successful both in their personal and professional lives. Others typically respond well to them so that they tend to have, from a young age, more self-confidence and assurance than their less good-looking peers.

Countless studies have shown that more attractive people are generally perceived as more intelligent, more honest, more successful, and more capable. The same studies have shown correlations between attractiveness and professional recognition, hiring decisions, promotions, and differences in salary levels.

Cosmetic surgery can make a difference to an individual's appearance and may indeed boost an individual's career and/or social status—especially when that individual is part of a creative or youth-driven industry. Moreover, quality of life in general can be dramatically improved by a cosmetic surgery procedure.

The same article described many ways in which the relief of a long-standing condition could significantly improve happiness levels. For a patient whose vision is improved by an eyelid lift, which removes the hooded part of the eyelid, the rewards are obvious. For a patient who has a breast reduction and experiences relief from long-standing daily pain, quality of life can also increase

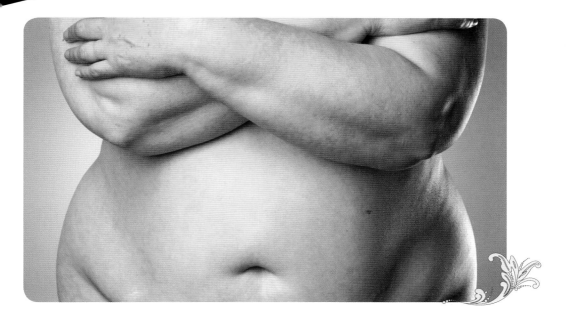

dramatically. For a patient who has 20lb (40kg) of loose hanging skin removed, it can mean feeling more comfortable, with increased levels of physical activity, which in turn can positively affect both mental and physical health.

One advance in cosmetic surgery, which reduces the risk of expectations being higher than likely outcomes, is the fact that new computer software means the surgeon can now show the patient an image of what he or she might expect to look like after surgery. The surgeon can take digital photographs of a patient and modify their image on the computer screen to show the reasonable outcome of any cosmetic procedure. The patient can also use this tool to show the doctor what they like or dislike about their current features or about

the potential outcome of the procedure.

The positive message for all would-be patients is certainly that cosmetic surgery administered by a top, certified surgeon can enhance not only looks but pleasure in life. But some consumer information websites point out that the success of cosmetic surgery is subjective, and that unsatisfactory outcomes such as excessive scarring or perceived asymmetry can devastate the patient.

At the end of the day, the potential rewards of cosmetic surgery are specific to the individual. Many patients say their only regret is that they didn't do it sooner. Others wholeheatedly wish they had never done it at all. Risk can be mitigated by doing your homework and becoming a very informed patient before any surgery.

# CHOOSING A
# COSMETIC SURGEON

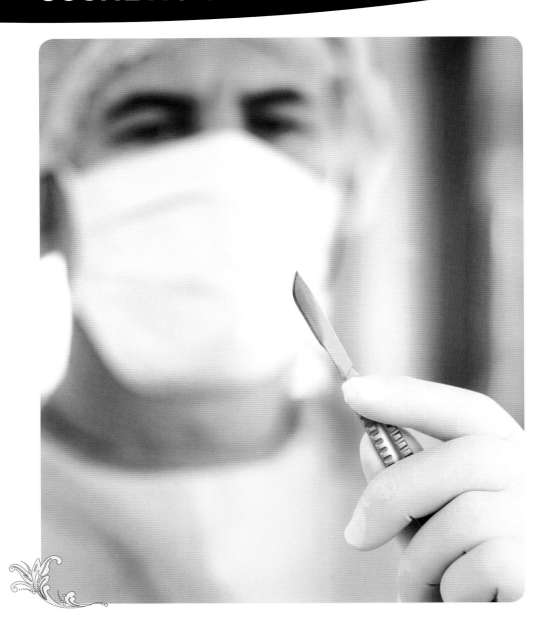

If, after a lot of careful self-evaluation and soul-searching, you have decided to have cosmetic surgery, then you will need to be prepared to make the next important step—finding a surgeon. Most cosmetic surgery involves a serious operation, and this can never be guaranteed to work perfectly. But the chances of anything going wrong are much less if your surgeon is qualified, ethical, and trustworthy.

## THE PLAN

In your quest for a cosmetic surgeon you will need to draw up a plan, which will cover all of the crucial factors involved in trusting someone with your body and your health.

## STAGE 1:
## DRAFT A LIST OF COSMETIC SURGEONS

Start to draft a list of cosmetic surgeons that you find; the best way to put together a list is to get recommendations from friends, colleagues, family, or people who have had a positive experience of a cosmetic surgeon. Personal referrals are highly valuable and extremely important—after all, a patient who has already used a cosmetic surgeon can give you the inside information on their skills, service, attitude, cost, and results. In the course of your research you are bound to come across some negative experiences of cosmetic surgeons from people you talk to. Try to keep these in perspective.

Call up the offices of advertised surgeons who seem promising, and find out what your options are through them; however don't choose a surgeon based solely on what you read on an advertisement or website. No matter how beautiful and polished a commercial may seem, it is not an indication of a surgeon's skill or expertise—there are many surgeons who do not advertise as they have enough patient referrals based purely on their reputation.

## STAGE 2:
## QUALIFY THE SURGEONS ON YOUR LIST

Qualifying a surgeon means that you have sufficient and satisfactory information about their certification, qualifications, and experience.

**Your cosmetic surgeon must have the following credentials:**

- Your surgeon must have completed medical school, and will be willing to show certificates
- Your surgeon must have completed a residency in plastic surgery
- Your surgeon must have a medical specialization
- Your surgeon must have hospital privileges for the procedure you want
- Your surgeon must be board-certified (vetted by their specialty board) as a Board Certified Plastic Surgeon or a Board Certified Cosmetic Surgeon
- Your surgeon must be a member of an

approved American Board of Medical Specialties Society, ideally the ASPS (American Society of Plastic Surgeons) or/and ASAPS (The American Society for Aesthetic Plastic Surgery)
- Your surgeon should have proven experience and demonstrated skill in plastic/cosmetic surgery.

## WHAT MAKES A COSMETIC SURGEON A "SPECIALIST"?

Medicine has so many different areas that one doctor could simply not know everything about all of them; therefore they choose areas of medicine to focus on. To become a surgical specialist a doctor must graduate from university, and then spend 4 years in medical school. Once that is complete the doctor must train "in residency"; this is a commitment that can last several years, whereby the doctor works at a hospital under the supervision of senior staff, allowing the doctor to gradually increase his experience and level of responsibility.

A plastic surgeon must complete 6–8 years of training after medical school. A facial plastic surgeon must complete 5–7 years of training after medical school, and a dermatologist normally trains for 3–5 years. When a doctor completes training they must apply to the state in which they work for a license to practice medicine. This is different from applying for board certification which, once given, is a specialty status recognized in all states.

## Clarifying "board-certified"

Passing "the boards" (a combination of written and oral exams) is crucial for all surgeons who have completed their training. Not everyone passes, and there are many good surgeons who are not board-certified. However, it is advised that you consult with a board-certified surgeon.

## STAGE 3:
## SCREENING SURGEONS—
## A TELEPHONE CHECKLIST

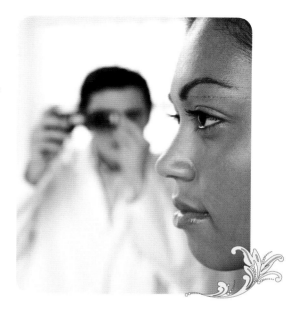

✔Check that the surgeon has a board certification approved by the ABMS (American Board of Medical Specialties). Does the certification and training include the procedure you are considering? For example, a facial plastic surgeon would be perfect for a facelift or a nose job, but would not necessarily be perfect for breast augmentation or tummy tuck surgery.

✔Ask the surgeon about his or her education and training; specifically, you may want to ask:
  • How long has the surgeon been in practice?
  • Where did the surgeon go to school?
  • How many years of surgical training did he or she complete?
  • Did he or she complete a residency in an ABMS-recognized specialty that would preferably include cosmetic surgery?
  • How many times does he or she perform the procedure you are interested in having per month?
  • What percentage of the surgeon's work is invasive or noninvasive?

  • What kind of post-operative care does the surgeon's practice offer?
  • How does the surgeon handle complications or post-surgical problems? And are there any associated costs?
  • What professional societies and organizations is the surgeon a member of?

✔Check that the surgeon operates in an accredited surgery center, hospital, or suite.

✔Ask what kinds of anesthesia options are available and who is the provider of anesthetic services; ask if the anesthetist is board-certified. If no anesthetist is available, ask who will perform the sedation—is it the surgeon or a member of the nursing team?

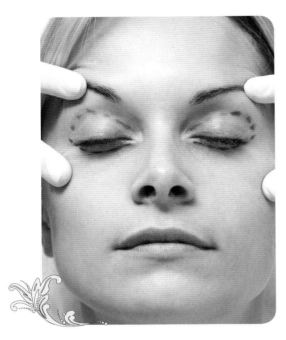

that you like. Trust should arise from faith in the surgeon's training, qualifications, certification, expertise, and proven results; likability stems from the personal characteristics that your surgeon displays such as communication skills, openness and honesty, kindness, and a good manner.

Even if the surgeon has a busy practice you shouldn't feel pressured into rushing your consultation; a good surgeon will allow you enough time to talk through all your questions. A consultation should not just be with a nurse or a patient co-ordinator; ideally it is the surgeon who will spend most of the time with you.

Ask about the surgeon's training and experience, even if you have already researched this information by telephone or on the Internet. A good surgeon should be willing to offer this information and should not be bothered by your questions.

Make sure the surgeon is listening to your objectives. Make your concerns and what you want to achieve clear—ensure that the surgeon has understood and suggests solutions that fit your concerns. If a surgeon understands your motivations this is beneficial to the whole process. For example, if you have undergone major weight-loss and want your self-confidence back, or if you are wanting to regain your pre-pregnancy shape, understanding what motivates you can create a good patient–surgeon bond, make the whole process

## STAGE 4:
## GETTING THE BEST FROM
## YOUR CONSULTATIONS

By this stage you should have gathered enough research and be armed with some essential information, as well as a shortlist of surgeons. Consultation visits are very important steps in your decision-making process, and so it is essential that you get as much as you can from them. The purpose of a consultation is to find a surgeon that you feel you can trust and

a lot more comfortable, and can even aid your recovery.

Make sure that you are satisfied with the answers to your questions. The surgeon should answer your questions in a way that is clear and comprehensible to you. You need to make sense of the information the surgeon gives you as this will help you in your final decision; don't be afraid to tell the surgeon you have not understood the answer to a particular question. Ideally a surgeon will equip you with some further reading materials or information to help you understand what you have spoken about during your consultation.

Be honest and open with your surgeon when he or she asks you about previous surgeries, your general medical history and current medical conditions, your lifestyle, any medications or drugs you use, consumption of alcohol, or use of tobacco. Being honest about these issues will not necessarily stop you having surgery but will help your surgeon and his medical team to care for you properly and prevent any issues prior to surgery and recovery.

Ask your surgeon about alternative solutions to surgery and their benefits. A good surgeon will always offer alternative options for you to consider, and one alternative may be not to have surgery at all. Ask to see "before and after" pictures. Photographs of previous work should give you a clear indication as to what kind of results the surgeon can achieve. A good surgeon's practice should have clear, recent, and well-organized photographs. Ask yourself: Am I impressed with the pictures? Are the people in the pictures

actual patients? (Don't be afraid to ask this question of the surgeon.) Do the results in the photographs look natural? Do I share the surgeon's aesthetic vision?

Ask how the surgeon and his team will help you prepare for surgery and recovery. For instance, how will they educate you in preparation for your procedure, and will they provide you with reading materials and take charge of communication for your care? Knowing how to prepare for surgery and recovery is vitally important.

Talk to former patients of the surgeon— most surgeons' practices can arrange for you to talk to one or more of their former

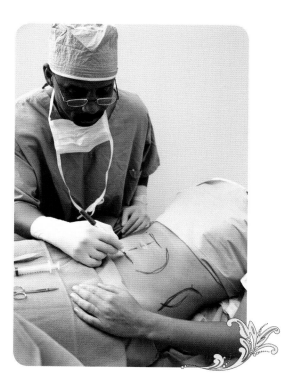

patients who have either had the same procedure that you are enquiring about, or a similar one. Good surgeons have lots of ex-patients who will be only too happy to talk about their experiences.

You should leave the consultation with a written quotation. This should include all the costs relating to your surgery. Make sure you also have information about any additional costs that you are likely to incur in the event of further surgery relating to a complication or a revision.

You should enter and leave a consultation feeling comfortable with both the surgeon and his staff. If the reception is cold, distant, and unfriendly by both the surgeon and staff then you are more likely to feel uncomfortable during your consultation. A good encounter should be positive and satisfying; feeling comfortable is crucial to achieving a good overall experience and not just a good surgical result.

## FINALLY...

Consulting with several surgeons is advised, however bear in mind that each surgeon will have a particular view of or approach to the cosmetic surgery procedure you want. Remember, you are looking for the best result for your body, so the latest techniques and innovations may not necessarily be the best option. Be aware of any surgeon who takes a one-size-fits-all approach; instead look for a surgeon who communicates well, shows willingness to consider other options, and shows consideration toward your objectives and needs.

By this stage, you should have a shortlist of one or two (or maybe more) surgeons. If you require a second consultation don't be afraid to schedule one; this will give you the opportunity to get answers to any outstanding questions you may have and a second chance to evaluate important issues.

Your final choice will involve both practical and emotional factors. Trust your intuition as well as your carefully gathered information to make a confident decision and move forward with your choice.

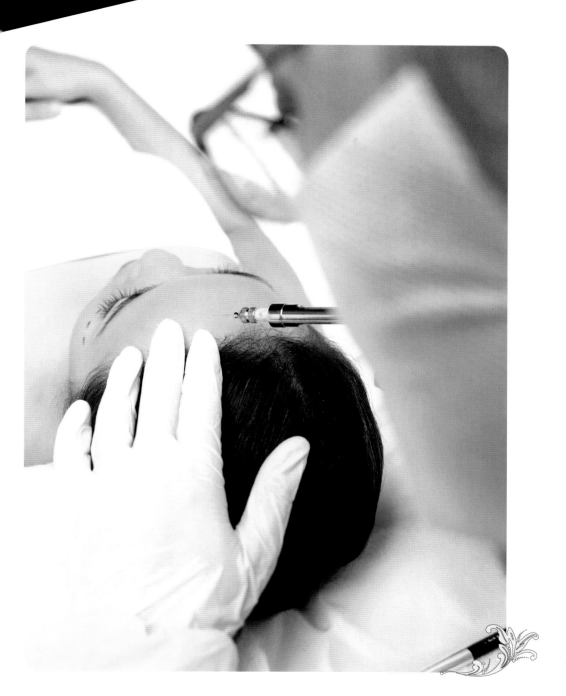

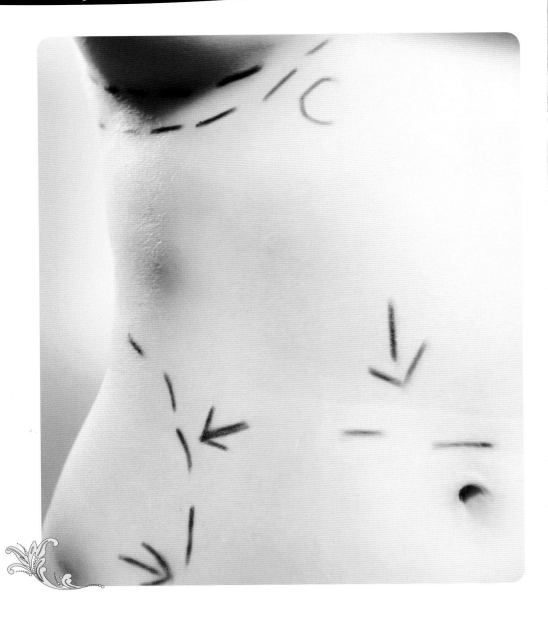

According to statistics from the American Society for Aesthetic Plastic Surgery, almost 10 million cosmetic surgical and nonsurgical procedures were performed in the United States in 2009. The society claims that the overall number of cosmetic procedures has increased by 147 percent since the tracking of the statistics first began. This clearly indicates that cosmetic surgery is growing in demand around the world. The most popular surgical procedures were breast augmentation, liposuction, rhinoplasty (nose surgery), eyelid surgery, and tummy tuck.

## 1. Breast augmentation

Breast augmentation aims to cosmetically enhance the size and shape of a woman's breasts using implants. It is performed for a number of reasons and these vary—some are cosmetic and some medical. In ever-increasing numbers, women are flocking to surgeons to have their breasts surgically enhanced with the use of silicone or saline implants: breast augmentation continues to be the single most popular cosmetic surgery procedure in the United States today, with 311,000 performed (2009 statistics). There are also other kinds of cosmetic breast surgery, including breast lifts and breast reductions, available as well.

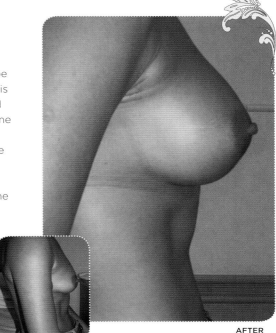

BEFORE

AFTER

## 2. Liposuction

Fat deposits that cannot be removed by diet or exercise usually occur in areas such as the chin, chest, stomach, sides, back, and thighs. Liposuction is a fat-removal procedure that aims to eradicate excessive stubborn fat from these hard-to-shift areas. Liposuction should be thought of as a sculpting procedure that can change the contours of your body or face. Some new nonsurgical or minimally invasive options for dealing with unwanted fat deposits, such as SmartLipo and acoustic wave therapy, have become increasingly popular. Over 283,000 liposuction procedures were performed in the U.S. in 2009.

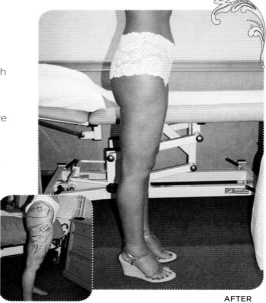

BEFORE

AFTER

## 3. Eyelid surgery

Eyelid surgery is a procedure to remove fat—usually along with excess skin and muscle—from the upper and lower eyelids. Eyelid surgery can lift drooping upper lids and reduce the puffy "bags" that form below your eyes. It can be done alone or in conjunction with other plastic facial surgery procedures such as a facelift. With the eyes being "the windows of the soul" it's no surprise to see this procedure on the most-wanted list.

AFTER

BEFORE

## 4. Tummy tuck

No amount of diet and exercise can get rid of excess skin. This is the reason for the popularity of the "tummy tuck." This procedure removes excess fat and skin from around the waist to leave a flatter lower-body profile and younger-looking abdomen. The procedure is most popular with people who have lost large amounts of weight and with women whose abdominal skin and muscles have been stretched beyond repair by pregnancy. While scarring is unavoidable, scars are almost always undetectable in a bikini, and many people are more than willing to trade this for the chance to have a flat stomach again.

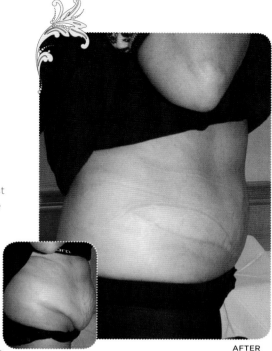

BEFORE

AFTER

## 5. Facelift

Due to the inevitable aging process, over time the reflection in your mirror starts to change... and if you are you not as excited about what you see in the mirror as you used to be then a cosmetic facelift could help you to rediscover your confidence and improve those little imperfections. A facelift, or the surgical removal of wrinkles, can reduce some of the more visible signs of aging. It smoothes the loose skin on your face and neck and tightens the underlying tissue. As a result, your face will appear firmer and fresher, in turn making you look younger.

AFTER

BEFORE

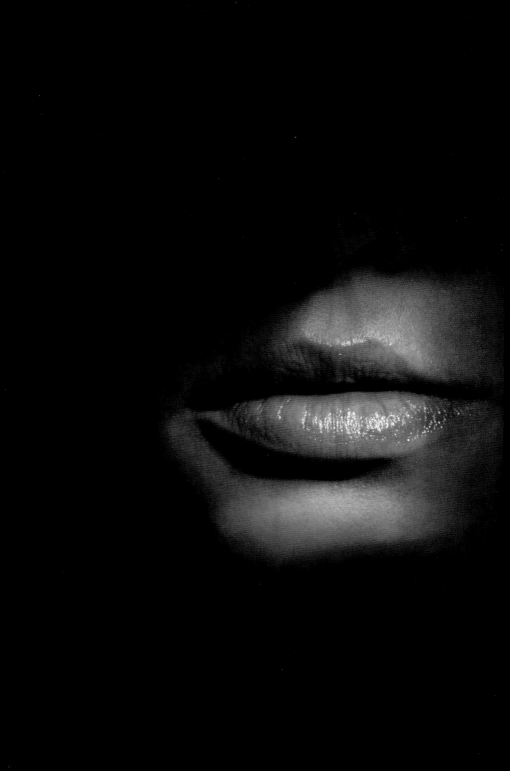

# CHAPTER TWO
# FACIAL COSMETIC SURGERY

# FACIAL COSMETIC SURGERY

*An overview*

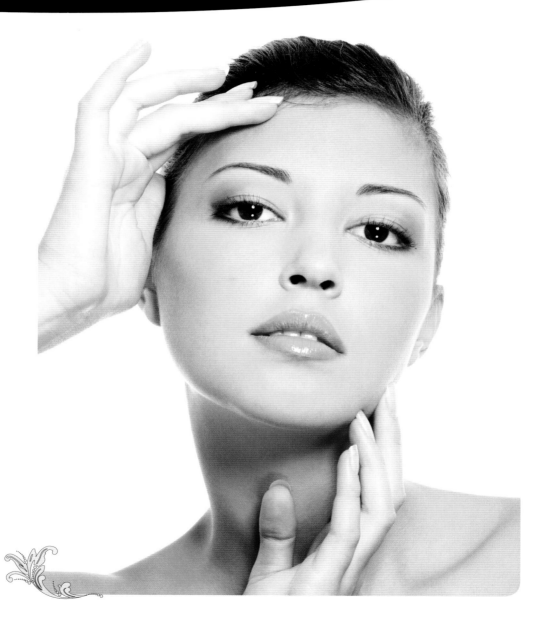

Cosmetic surgery of the face and neck is generally undergone either to give the face a more youthful appearance or to improve the shape and contour of facial features such as the nose, eyes, cheeks, chin, brow, ears, or neck. It is extremely popular among those who wish to hit back at the aging process, but also in instances where correction may be made to, for example, prominent noses or ears. Consequently, there are many plastic surgery procedures in line with these demands.

You may be a suitable candidate for a facial cosmetic surgery procedure if you are unhappy with how the aging process is affecting your face and neck, or if you have a congenital deformity that needs to be corrected to enhance your appearance. You must also be in good physical and emotional health and have realistic expectations about the outcome of your surgery.

After you have located a reputable board-certified cosmetic surgeon (see pages 28–35), you will have an initial consultation to discuss the changes that you would like to make. The surgeon will explain the options available for your individual requirements, the steps of the procedure that you desire, the different types of facial plastic surgery available, the risks, side effects, complications and limitations, and the costs.

The surgeon will also explain how your chosen individual facial surgical procedure varies in time and technique, as well as providing recovery and healing information.

Some of the most popular facial cosmetic surgery procedures sought by patients include: neck lift, rhinoplasty (nose surgery), otoplasty (ear surgery or ear pinning), lip augmentation, lip enhancement, facelift surgery, blepharoplasty (eyelid surgery and eye bag surgery), chin surgery, and cheek implants—these are all covered in greater detail in this chapter.

If you're considering facial surgery, the following information will provide you with a good introduction to the procedures available. For more detailed information about how these procedures may help you, you should consult a board-certified facial surgeon.

# FACELIFT SURGERY
## *Rhytidectomy*

### WHY HAVE FACELIFT SURGERY?

Facelift surgery (technically known as rhytidectomy) can make you look younger and fresher by improving the appearance of your face. The aim of a facelift is to make you look "good for your age," with a natural, more youthful appearance. A facelift procedure is likely to be successful if you have good skin tone—if your skin has not lost its elasticity, and moves and stretches easily.

## *What is the procedure?*

**Your face is made up of layers of bone, muscle, fascia, fat, and skin. During the natural aging process, the muscles lose their tone, and the fascia (which holds everything together) slackens. The fat around the lower half of the face may drop down and form a "jowly" look, causing deep wrinkles and folds. The cell-renewal cycle shortens, and the skin is less able to regenerate and loses elasticity. A facelift will improve the sagging areas that have lost their tone, but cannot remove permanent perpendicular wrinkles on the upper and lower lips, or on the forehead.**

## *Am I a candidate for facelift surgery?*

Facelift surgery can be an effective way to improve the appearance and boost self-confidence, but it is not for everyone. Patients whose skin is still relatively supple, and who are in good overall health achieve the best results. Some patients combine facelift surgery with other procedures, such as a neck lift or brow lift. Patients with realistic expectations are more often pleased with the results.

The majority of patients who undergo facelift surgery do so between the ages of 40 and 60, though patients in their 70s and 80s have had this surgery successfully.

A facelift will normally not be necessary for people under 40, though patients with premature facial aging or who have had significant weight loss may benefit earlier.

**If you are concerned by any of the following, you could benefit:**
- Sagging in the mid face
- Deep creases below the lower eyelids
- Deep creases running from the nose to the corners of the mouth
- "Jowls" caused by loss of muscle tone in the lower part of the face
- Displaced fat.

## WHAT TO EXPECT FROM A CONSULTATION WITH A FACELIFT SURGEON

During this consultation a surgeon will assess your physical and emotional health and discuss your goals and objectives for the facelift. You will also be asked for information about your previous surgeries, past and present medical conditions, and treatments you have received; you will also be asked to provide information about any medications you are taking.

The surgeon will also carry out a physical evaluation in which your bone structure will be assessed as well as the thickness, texture, and elasticity of your skin. A surgeon will also assess the severity of wrinkles and folds. Your hairline will be examined to determine where incisions could be placed. All of these factors will be considered in developing your surgical plan.

The surgeon will also discuss the types of facelift procedures available to decide on the one that best suits your individual requirements, as well as discussing the possibility of additional procedures that can be performed along with a facelift.

**Other procedures frequently combined with facelift surgery include:**
- Forehead lift to correct lines or furrows in the brow
- Eyelid surgery to eliminate drooping upper eyelids or bags beneath the eyes
- Nose reshaping
- Skin treatments such as injectable fillers, chemical peels, or laser resurfacing to minimize fine lines and wrinkles.

## Technical advances

New procedures have been developed over the last 15–20 years, including the SMAS facelift, the extended SMAS facelift, and the deep plane facelift.

**SMAS facelift:** The SMAS (Superficial Musculo Aponeurotic System) facelift is a deeper facelift that pulls back the muscles and connective tissues in the neck and face, and repositions the fat and muscles on the cheekbones.

**Extended SMAS facelift:** The extended SMAS facelift is the most popular facelift in the U.S. It is much like the SMAS facelift, except that it also focuses on correcting the middle of the face by extending farther toward the nose.

**Deep plane facelift:** The deep plane facelift begins with an incision in the scalp for the brow lift. Incisions are also made in the lower eyelid and inside the mouth. This facelift is better suited to younger patients because it does not involve surgery of the neck. Unfortunately, it takes a while for the swelling to go down, so results of the facelift are not always noticeable until 3-6 months after surgery.

# The basic procedure

The technique chosen for your facelift surgery will depend on your surgeon's preferences in relation to your features as well as your desired results and personal objectives.

There are many variations on the basic facelift procedure, however, the incision is typically made in the natural contour behind your ear, and then extends around the earlobe and back into the hairline. The incision can normally be concealed by your hair or with makeup; in some cases there may also be a small incision hidden beneath your chin.

It is through these incisions that your surgeon will free the facial skin from the underlying tissues and pull it upward and backward. Any excess skin is removed; in some cases deeper tissues can also be repositioned to restore a more youthful contour to the face.

If you have fatty tissue in the chin area a surgeon may also make an incision and remove that as well as smoothing out any corded underlying muscle in the neck.

## Preparing for facelift surgery

When the date for your surgical procedure has been established, your surgeon will provide you with specific instructions for the days prior to your surgery and also after the surgery. Such instructions may include:

- Avoiding medications that could complicate surgery or recovery

- Ceasing smoking for a period of time before and after your facelift procedure
- Arranging for special care and help after your surgery
- Letting your hair grow sufficiently long to cover your incisions while they are healing.

## 1. ANESTHESIA

Facelift surgery normally takes anything from 2–3 hours and is performed under general anesthesic; there are some forms of minimally invasive facelift procedures that can be performed under local anesthetic and sedation (also known as "twilight anesthesia").

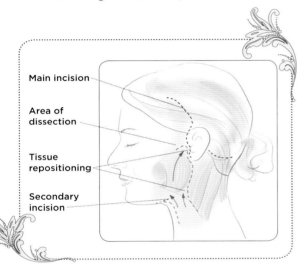

Main incision

Area of dissection

Tissue repositioning

Secondary incision

## 2. THE INCISIONS

There are various choices when you have a facelift and the incisions you have depend very much on the facelift procedure you and your surgeon have chosen to best suit your needs.

## 3. THE SUTURES

Non-absorbable sutures or skin adhesives on the incisions on the face and small metal staples around the hairline are used to close the facelift incisions. Once the surgery has been completed, the face and the entire head will be bandaged as loosely as possible in order to reduce bruising and swelling.

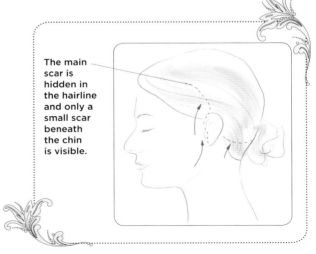

The main scar is hidden in the hairline and only a small scar beneath the chin is visible.

# Recovery and healing

Facelift recovery times vary from patient to patient, and smokers take longer to heal. You may need pain relief to help with any discomfort as the anesthetic wears off. If you need them, you can take over-the-counter painkillers such as paracetamol or ibuprofen. (Follow the instructions in the patient information leaflet that comes with the medicine and ask your pharmacist for advice.)

You will need to arrange for someone to drive you home when you are ready to go. You should also arrange to have a friend or relative stay with you for at least the first 24 hours. Your nurse will give you some advice about caring for your wounds and a date for a follow-up appointment before you go home.

The swelling will be at its worst 2–3 days after facelift surgery; sleeping upright in bed supported by pillows and applying ice packs will help to reduce the swelling. Rest as much as possible for the first week, keep your incision sites dry, and avoid closed-neck clothing to prevent contact with your head and face.

Some numbness, swelling, and even discoloration of the skin is likely to occur, lasting for up to 2 weeks after the surgery.

After 5–10 days your stitches will be removed, and a few days later you should start to see the results of the facelift. From 5–14 days after the facelift procedure you will start to look and feel better and will be able to take gentle walks and do light housework. Visible swelling and bruising should go down after 4–6 weeks—avoid any strenuous activity during this time. You will probably feel numbness in your face for a few weeks, which is caused by the stress put on the nerves during and after the facelift operation.

It may take several months for the swelling to fully dissipate and up to 6 months for incision lines to mature. Maintaining or adopting a healthy lifestyle and wearing a high-SPF sun screen whenever you go out will help to extend the results of your facelift. You will see the end result of your facelift approximately 6–9 months after your facelift operation.

## FACTS
### FACELIFT

| | |
|---|---|
| **Description** | The skin of the face is stretched back and up to give a fresher, more youthful apperance. |
| **Length of surgery** | 2–3 hours |
| **In/outpatient** | Inpatient |
| **Anesthesia** | General |
| **Back to work in...** | 4 weeks |
| **Back to the gym in...** | 6 weeks |
| **Treatment frequency** | One or more times as desired |
| **Risks** | • Soreness, swelling, and bruising—this can last up to a month<br>• Scarring—this usually fades over the course of a year, but won't completely disappear<br>• Raised hairline in front of, and behind, your ears<br>• Bleeding<br>• Reaction to the anesthetic<br>• Infection<br>• Deep vein thrombosis<br>• Damage of facial nerves resulting in muscle weakness<br>• Raised keloid scarring<br>• Asymmetrical ears<br>• Dissatisfaction with results<br>• Hematoma (a collection of blood under the skin that may require surgery to stop the bleeding and to drain the area)<br>• Hair loss around the scars |
| **Duration of results** | 5–10 years |

# EYELID SURGERY
*Blepharoplasty*

## WHY HAVE EYELID SURGERY?

Eyelid surgery, technically known as blepharoplasty, is a cosmetic surgical procedure that can improve the appearance of the eyes to create a more youthful appearance. Eyelid surgery can be performed on the upper or lower eyelids, or both.

## What is the procedure?

**Eyelid surgery can improve the loose or sagging skin that creates folds or disturbs the natural contour of the upper eyelids; this can in some cases lead to impaired vision. Eyelid surgery can also remove fatty deposits in the upper eyelids that can make a person's eyelids look puffy and swollen.**

**For the lower eyelids surgery can remove bags under the eyes, correct droopiness of the eyelids, and remove excess skin and fine wrinkles of the eyelid.**

## Am I a candidate for a eyelid surgery?

People over 35 years of age are normally candidates for eyelid surgery, though younger people may undergo blepharoplasty if they have large under-eye bags. More than half of all blepharoplasty patients are over 50 years old.

**Eyelid surgery may be suitable for you if you are bothered by:**
- Puffiness or bags under the lower lids
- Excess skin and wrinkles on the lower lids
- Loose folds of skin on the upper eyelids.

Eye surgery is usually performed on adult men and women who have healthy facial tissue and muscles, are in good health physically and emotionally, and have realistic expectations about what eyelid surgery can and cannot achieve.

However, there are reasons why some people are not good candidates for lower eyelid surgery, even if they fulfill some of the criteria above. There are some medical conditions which increase the risk of complications from lower eyelid surgery.

## WHAT TO EXPECT FROM A CONSULTATION WITH AN EYELID SURGEON

The surgeon will ask you about your health during the consultation. Make sure you tell him or her about any medical condition you have so that together you can make the best choice prior to surgery; be as candid as possible with your surgeon to ensure that your operation proceeds safely and successfully.

**Your surgeon will evaluate your general health; therefore expect to be asked about:**

- Your objectives and reasons for wanting eyelid surgery and your desired outcome
- Medical conditions, drug allergies, and previous medical treatments
- Previous surgeries
- Current use of medications, vitamins, supplements, and possibly alcohol, tobacco, and drugs.

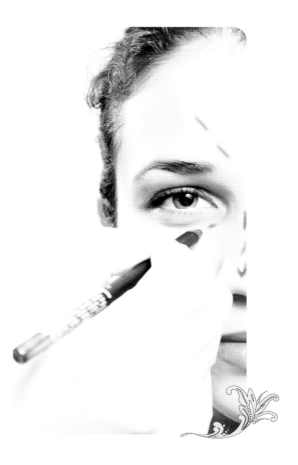

### Those at risk from eye surgery include people with:

- Hyperthyroidism
- High blood pressure (hypertension)
- "Dry eye" or problems with the tear ducts
- Graves' disease
- Glaucoma
- Detached retina
- Cardiovascular disease
- Diabetes.

If you are considering eyelid surgery but are being treated for or are concerned that you may be suffering from any of these conditions, discuss your concerns with your own doctor beforehand.

# The basic procedure

## 1. ANESTHESIA

Your face will be swabbed with disinfectant and draped in sterile sheets. The blepharoplasty surgeon will measure the exact amount of skin to be removed and mark this on the skin on your eyelids and around your eyes. The surgeon will then administer local anesthesia, starting at the outer aspect of the lower eyelids and continuing toward the inner lower eyelids.

## 2. THE INCISIONS

The surgeon will make incisions along the marks made on your skin, so that the scars will be hidden in natural creases. There are two incision options:

- Inside the eyelid (if you only need excess fatty tissue removed, not skin). The tissues are separated to obtain access to the fat pockets in the lower eyelid. The pockets of fat are exposed and a series of surgical instruments are used to remove, or tease out, the fat.

- Alternatively, the surgeon may operate on your lower eyelid by making an incision outside the eyelid. An incision is made just underneath the lid margin and the skin is gently pulled back to allow the surgeon to dissect the underlying fat pockets. The surgeon will gently press on the eye to better expose the fat that will be removed, then remove the fat and the excess skin.

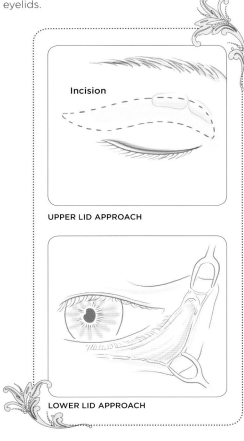

Incision

UPPER LID APPROACH

LOWER LID APPROACH

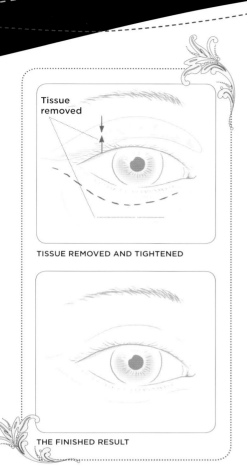

Tissue removed

**TISSUE REMOVED AND TIGHTENED**

**THE FINISHED RESULT**

**Eyelid surgery scars are not visible as they are concealed in the natural creases around the eye.**

### 3. THE SUTURES

If the incision was made inside the eyelid, sutures may or may not be used, depending on your surgeon's preference. If the incision was made outside the eyelid, the wounds are closed with fine sutures which will be removed after 3–5 days.

Small adhesive strips are placed over the sutures, and the surgeon will probably lubricate your eyes with ointment and may apply a compression bandage.

Your eyelids may feel tight and sore as the anesthesia wears off, and your surgeon will prescribe pain medication to make you more comfortable.

### 4. THE RESULTS

You will need to keep your head elevated for several days after the procedure and use cold compresses to reduce swelling and bruising. The extent and severity of bruising varies from patient to patient. It is worst during the first week, but should clear up after 2–4 weeks.

Before you leave the hospital or clinic, you will be shown how to clean your eyes, which may be sticky for a week or so. Your doctor may recommend eye drops, as your eyelids will probably feel dry at first and may itch or burn.

In the first few weeks after your operation, your eyes may feel "teary," you may feel sensitive to light, and you may also experience blurring or double vision. The stitches will be removed about a week after lower eyelid surgery. Once they're removed the swelling and bruising around your eyes will subside, and your new look will begin to emerge.

## Preparing for eyelid surgery

Prior to surgery you may be asked to:

- Have lab tests or a medical evaluation
- Take certain medications or adjust any medications you may be taking
- Stop smoking
- Avoid medications such as aspirin, anti-inflammatories, and herbal supplements.

You will also receive special instructions regarding what you should do the night before surgery and on the morning of surgery, and will be given instructions and information regarding the use of anesthesia for your surgical procedure.

## Recovery and healing

Eyelid swelling and bruising are common post-operative side effects in the first few days after surgery, though these can last up to 2 weeks. A rest regime, sleeping with your head elevated, and using ice compresses applied with pressure can all speed up the healing process.

You will be able to wear makeup again after 2 weeks, and return to sports and physical activities after 3–4 weeks. You must avoid strong sunlight during your recovery time, as the skin around the eyes will be even more sensitive than usual. You will need to wear a sunscreen with a very high SPF, sunglasses, and hats for 6–8 weeks.

## Tips for a speedy recovery:

- Sleep propped up on pillows to reduce swelling and bruising
- Avoid bending forward for a few days
- Carefully cleanse around your eyes and use the ointment prescribed by your surgeon
- Don't wear contact lenses for at least 2 weeks
- Don't drive until your eyes have stopped watering and your vision has returned to normal.

# FACTS
## EYELID SURGERY

| | |
|---|---|
| **Description** | A cosmetic surgical procedure that can improve the appearance of the eyes to give a more youthful look. |
| **Length of surgery** | 1–3 hours |
| **In/outpatient** | Inpatient or outpatient |
| **Anesthesia** | Local or general |
| **Back to work in...** | Several days |
| **Back to the gym in...** | 3–4 weeks |
| **Treatment frequency** | One or more times, as desired |
| **Risks** | • Soreness, swelling, and bruising around the eyes<br>• Sticky, dry, and itchy eyes<br>• Watery eyes<br>• Sensitivity to light<br>• Double or blurred vision<br>• Scarring<br>• Hematoma (a collection of blood under the skin that may require surgery to stop the bleeding and to drain the area)<br>• Sensation disturbances (usually temporary)<br>• Damage to the surface of the eyeball<br>• Sunken or uneven appearance<br>• Infection<br>• Pigmentation changes<br>• Poor healing of the skin—most likely to affect smokers<br>• Allergic reaction to the anesthesia |
| **Duration of results** | Long-lasting |

# CHIN SURGERY
## *Genioplasty*

## *What is the procedure?*

**This procedure can range from injecting temporary soft tissue filler to implanting a silicone or Porex chin implant, to having a full genioplasty. Chin augmentation is often used in conjunction with other forms of cosmetic surgery.**

## WHY HAVE CHIN SURGERY?

Chin augmentation is a common procedure intended to reshape or change the size of the chin. The procedure is often sought by patients with a prominent nose, a weak chin due to congenital deficiency, age-related bone resorption, or facial trauma. Patients normally consider chin surgery if they wish to create a more balanced facial appearance.

## *Am I a candidate for genioplasty?*

First and foremost, you should be in good health, must not have any active diseases or pre-existing medical conditions, and should have realistic expectations of the outcome of your surgery. You must be mentally and emotionally stable to undergo any cosmetic procedure and chin surgery is no exception. You'll need patience to deal with the healing period.

Only a qualified cosmetic surgeon can determine your suitability for surgery after going over your medical history, and examining your facial structure and skin.

### WHAT TO EXPECT FROM A CONSULTATION WITH A CHIN SURGEON

After the surgeon has examined you and taken your medical history, you will have the opportunity to discuss the various options available for your chin surgery procedure. Your surgeon will individualize the specific chin augmentation procedure to suit your desires and exact chin deficiencies. Aesthetic genioplasty is typically performed to add size and contour to a receding chin; the extent of the procedure varies. Patients with a normal dental bite, but a weak or receding chin, are the best candidates for genioplasty.

### At the consultation you may discuss:
- Your goals and objectives for the surgery
- The options available to you depending on your individual requirements
- The likely outcome of the procedure
- The risks, potential complications, and side effects.

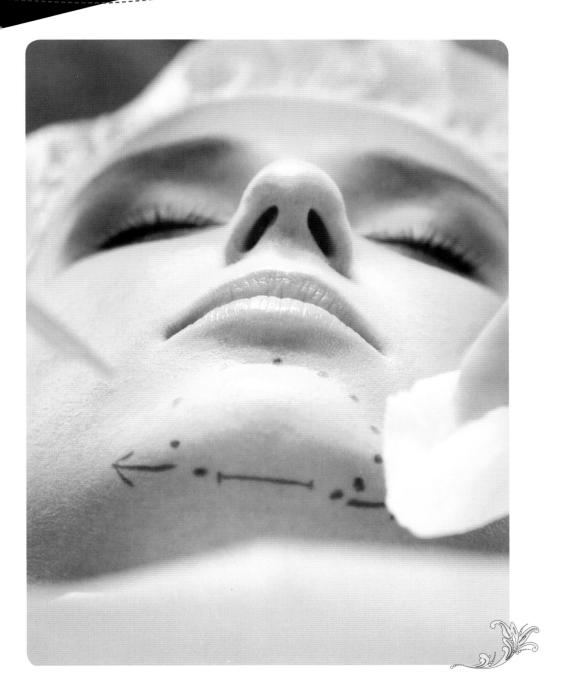

# The basic procedure

There are two approaches to genioplasty. In most patients a chin augmentation can be performed using a chin implant (see below). This is a simple procedure where an implant is placed either through the mouth or through a small incision under the chin. The patient can almost immediately resume normal activities. There is only minimal discomfort with this procedure, which takes about 30 minutes to 1 hour to perform.

However, it may be best to move the chin bone (see opposite). In this technique, the surgeon will make an incision inside the mouth to gain access. The lower portion of the separated bone is moved forward and wired in position. The incision in the mouth is then closed with sutures. Since surgery is performed through an internal incision, there is no visible scarring.

If you are having an injectable, a surgical team, general anesthesia, and operating room will not generally be needed, so this type of procedure can be much lower in price than the surgical option. It is advisable to discuss both types of chin augmentation with your surgeon and establish whether you will need "touch-ups" in the future to maintain your desired chin shape if you do choose an injectable treatment.

## 1. ANESTHESIA

The surgeon will have taken x-rays of your chin to determine which part to work on, and which approach to use. This will determine whether general anesthesia or local anesthesia with sedation will be used.

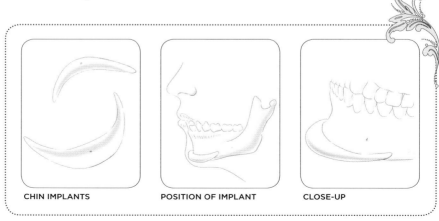

CHIN IMPLANTS      POSITION OF IMPLANT      CLOSE-UP

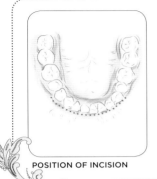

POSITION OF INCISION

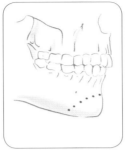

POSITION OF BONE CUT

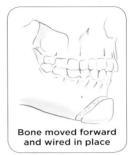

Bone moved forward and wired in place

NEW BONE POSITION

## 2. THE INCISIONS AND AUGMENTATION

A small incision is made in the natural crease under the chin or inside the mouth. The advantage of incisions inside the mouth is that visible scars will not be created; however, the chance of infection is increased, especially if plaque or other oral bacteria is present. You will discuss incision placement with your doctor before surgery. After the incision, the surgeon stretches the tissue to form a pocket to fit the customized implant. After the implant (made of silicone, Teflon, or Dacron) is inserted, the surgeon molds it to the desired contour then fixes the implant in place with a suture or places it beneath the jawbone's fibrous protective layer.

If the chin size is being reduced, the surgeon, after making a similar incision, sculpts the bone of the chin to change the appearance. The two types most commonly performed are sliding genioplasty or chin osteotomy. For the first, an incision is made through the bottom lip and the surgeon cuts the bone with an electric saw.

Having slid the bone into its new position, the bones are wired into place. The second type involves the removal of excess bone. This surgery is complicated and usually takes about 90 minutes.

## 3. THE SUTURES

The cut is closed with dissolvable stitches inside the mouth, or regular stitches under the chin, and a bandage is applied. Sutures inside the mouth will dissolve after about 10 days, and sutures outside the mouth are removed after the same period.

## 4. THE RESULTS

The results are immediately obvious, although you may think that the implant is too big at first because of swelling. The finished result is not apparent until about 6–8 weeks after the chin augmentation procedure. The scar may appear prominent for a few weeks after your surgery and will then start to fade. Some people, especially smokers, scar more than others.

# Recovery and healing

While recovery from chin augmentation surgery is quick compared to other types of facial cosmetic surgery procedures, there will be some restrictions on your activities for a short period after your surgery. After your chin augmentation procedure, you will be required to wear a protective covering over your chin for 2–4 days. You will experience some bruising and swelling around your chin and neck, and a relatively small amount of pain. Take the painkillers prescribed to you if you need them.

You can also expect some numbness, soreness, and tenderness which can last as long as 3 months. You will probably have some difficulty with smiling and talking, but this is only temporary and you should feel better in a few days.

You will probably have to stick to a liquid diet for a day or so, and you can resume light activity the day of the surgery. Even though you may not feel like it, your surgeon will more than likely advise you to walk and move around as soon as you are able. If you do not, you may develop clots or hold fluid (swelling, edema) a lot longer.

After surgery, you will need to have someone drive you home. Your surgeon should give you detailed instructions on your post-operative care, including instructions on brushing your teeth and rinsing your mouth in such a way as to avoid irritating the area. Stitches placed in the mouth will dissolve in 10 days to 2 weeks. Non-dissolving sutures will be removed during one of your follow-up visits.

Most chin augmentation patients are ready to resume normal activities after a few days, but avoid contact sports and any activity which might cause an impact to your face for 3 or 4 weeks. Also avoid any activities that require you to wear a helmet or chin-strap for the same period of time.

## Tips for a speedy recovery:

- Use ice packs or cold compresses on the area, but don't hold for too long in the same place
- Keep your head elevated when resting or sleeping
- Eat soft foods that do not require vigorous chewing, or drink protein shakes for a day or so
- Take any medications that your plastic surgeon recommends, including pain medications, mouth rinses, ointments, or salves
- Take your temperature regularly, as a raised temperature can indicate an infection.

# FACTS
## CHIN SURGERY

| | |
|---|---|
| **Description** | Procedure to reshape or increase the size of the chin for better projection and appearance. |
| **Length of surgery** | 1–3 hours |
| **In/outpatient** | Outpatient |
| **Anesthesia** | Local or general |
| **Back to work in...** | A few days |
| **Back to the gym in...** | 3–4 weeks |
| **Treatment frequency** | Once (or more with injectable fillers) |
| **Risks** | • Temporary swelling<br>• Bruising and tenderness<br>• Numbness of the lip and chin<br>• Weakening of the mouth<br>• Slow healing<br>• Infection<br>• Excessive bleeding<br>• An allergic reaction to the anesthesia<br>• Hematoma—a collection of blood under the skin<br>• Seroma—collection of fluid around the chin implant or incision<br>• Blood clots<br>• Damage to the teeth<br>• Extrusion—the chin implant works its way back up to the skin's surface<br>• Capsular contracture<br>• Asymmetry<br>• Nerve damage<br>• Bone erosion |
| **Duration of results** | Permanent (except for injectable fillers) |

# EAR SURGERY
## *Otoplasty*

### WHY HAVE EAR SURGERY?

Otoplasty, pinback, or ear reduction surgery can help protruding ears. Ears stick out from the head and when they excessively protrude, the deformity can be very disturbing. Otoplasty is the term for a number of operations to resculpt and reshape the ear.

## What is the procedure?

**Otoplasty can be performed on people at any age. Either a single ear or both ears may be involved. Techniques vary among otoplasty surgeons and from patient to patient. Factors that may influence the choice of technique include the general anatomy of the ears, the extent of the ear cartilage, excessive skin in the surrounding area, or the level of deformity in other areas of the ears.**

## Am I a candidate for an otoplasty procedure?

You may be a good candidate if you have:

- Protruding ear(s)
- Large ear(s)
- Abnormally shaped ear(s)

As long as you are in good health, there is no upper age limit for otoplasty surgery. However, there are reasons why some people are not good candidates for otoplasty, even if they fulfill the criteria above. Some medical conditions increase the risk of complications from ear surgery, including high blood pressure (hypertension), thyroid problems, and diabetes.

### WHAT TO EXPECT FROM A CONSULTATION WITH AN EAR SURGEON

The surgeon will likely ask you if you have any history of developmental disorders or hearing problems. The ears will be examined and compared to each other and to "normal" guidelines, and then they will be measured. The particular technique that your surgeon recommends will depend on the nature of the problem and your aesthetic goals and objectives. As every patient is different, not everyone will achieve the same results from ear surgery. Your ear surgeon will select the surgical technique that he or she feels will obtain the best outcome for you.

# The basic procedure

## 1. ANESTHESIA

Your surgeon will draw marks on the skin of your ear prior to the operation to mark the incision site(s). If you are nervous, you may be given a tranquilizer such as Valium to calm you down. An intravenous line will be placed in your arm or hand, and the sedation is administered through this line. (In patients under 14 years old, a general anesthetic is administered.) For your safety during the operation, various monitors are used to check your heart, blood pressure, pulse, and the amount of oxygen circulating in your blood.

## 2. THE INCISIONS AND RESHAPING/REMOVAL OF CARTILAGE AND/OR SKIN

There are two common otoplasty techniques. In the first, the surgeon finds the most inconspicuous site on the back of the ear to make the incision. Once the incision is made, the surgeon sculpts the exposed ear cartilage and repositions it closer to the head. The surgeon may use permanent sutures to help the cartilage stay in position. If necessary for the patient, the ear surgeon will remove excessive cartilage to improve the final appearance of the ear.

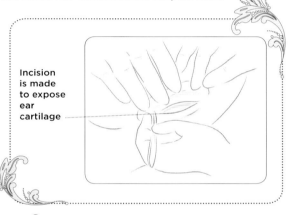

Incision is made to expose ear cartilage

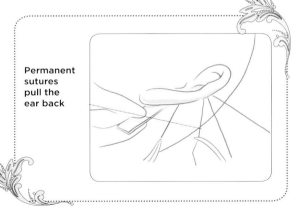

Permanent sutures pull the ear back

In the second technique, skin is removed, a small file is passed to the front of the ear to gently score the cartilage, and the ear cartilage is folded back. After making markings in the cartilage, stitches are placed through the back of the ear cartilage without going all the way through the front of the ear. After a series of these permanent sutures are placed, they are tied down, creating a folding

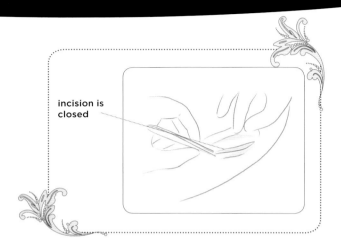

incision is
closed

of the ear to create a normal, more aesthetically pleasing, contour. There is no cartilage removed in this technique. At this point, the bowl (concha) of the ear can be tilted back if necessary, and any adjustments to the earlobe are made. The skin is then closed with absorbable sutures that will dissolve within 7 days, or with removable sutures that will be removed in 5–7 days.

## 3. THE RESULTS

When the surgery is complete, you will be taken into the recovery area where you will continue to be closely monitored. Tell your nurse or the surgeon if the dressings feel too tight. You should only feel a little discomfort from the ear surgery, especially if the ears are in a head dressing. Your ears will be swollen, bruised, and numb for 2 or 3 days after your ear surgery. Healing takes at least 6 weeks to be complete, and longer for all of the fine details of the ears to return to their normal appearance. You will normally be allowed home after a short period of observation, although some patients may stay overnight in the hospital or surgical facility.

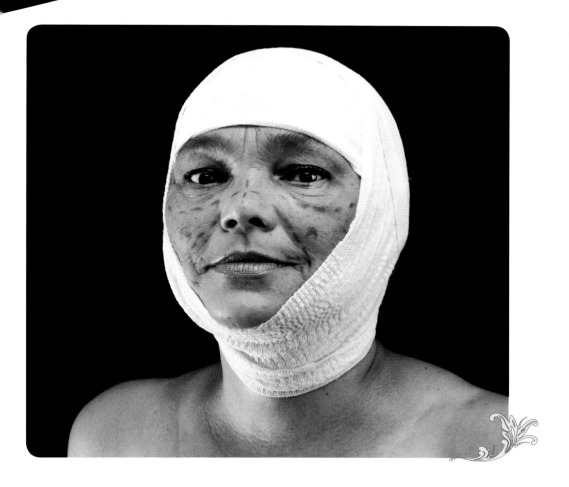

## Preparing for otoplasty

Your otoplasty surgeon will give you specific instructions on how to prepare for ear surgery, including guidelines on eating and drinking, smoking, and taking or avoiding certain vitamins and medications. Listening to this advice and following these instructions will help your surgery to go more smoothly and will help to reduce the risk of possible ear surgery side effects and complications.

# Recovery and healing

Otoplasty recovery times will vary from patient to patient and according to the extent of the ear surgery performed. Healing time after ear surgery depends on a patient's physical and emotional health and their response to surgery. Patients with a history of medical problems such as scarring or circulation problems, and patients who smoke may experience a longer healing time. The rate also depends on the quality of a patient's aftercare, and whether or not any complications are experienced. You must not take aspirin or certain anti-inflammatory medications.

After the procedure, your head is wrapped in a thick bandage, which helps to maintain the new position of the ears, protects them, and aids the healing process.

You will need to return to the surgeon's office within the first few days to have the bandage changed for a lighter one.

Most adult patients return to normal activity within 3 days of otoplasty surgery. More complicated procedures may require a longer recovery time. Children can return to normal activities in 7 days, but must be watched in playful activities for at least 3 weeks to avoid damage to the healing ears. For both adults and children, ears should not be bent for at least a month.

For the first several days you should maintain head elevation as much as possible. Sleep propped up on pillows to help to reduce the swelling caused by your ear surgery. Mild swelling may persist for many weeks in some patients. Bruising typically disappears within 7–10 days and stitches are usually removed within a week of otoplasty surgery.

You should only experience mild to moderate pain following your ear surgery, which is usually controlled by prescribed pain medication. You may also be prescribed an antibiotic to prevent or treat any infection. You will need to keep the dressing clean and dry, but you will be able to shower after the dressings are removed 3 or 4 days after the procedure. Your ears will be swollen, bruised, and numb, and may look a little irregular from the pressure of the dressings. Don't worry about this— it is very uncommon for ears to be perfectly symmetrical.

After surgery, you may be instructed to wear a gauze dressing or bandage for a few days or up to several weeks to ensure that your ears heal in their new, corrected position. A wide elastic hairband is worn at night to cover the ears and prevent them from bending during sleep. Avoid straining, bending, and lifting in the days following your otoplasty.

## FACTS
### EAR SURGERY

| | |
|---|---|
| **Description** | Ear reduction surgery to help the appearance of protruding ears. |
| **Length of surgery** | Local, or general for under-18s |
| **In/outpatient** | Outpatient |
| **Anesthesia** | Local or general |
| **Back to work in...** | 7–10 days |
| **Back to the gym in...** | 10 days |
| **Treatment frequency** | Once |
| **Risks** | • Temporary discomfort and numbness<br>• Headaches<br>• Swelling<br>• Bruising<br>• Asymmetry<br>• Itching or numbness at the incision line<br>• Hematoma<br>• Infection in the cartilage area<br>• Changes in sensation<br>• Scarring<br>• Blood clot on the ear<br>• Allergic reactions to the anesthesia<br>• Damage to underlying structures<br>• Need for revision surgery<br>• Unsatisfactory results<br>• Sutures may be visible or may break allowing for partial or complete recurrence of the protrusion and/or loss of the ear fold, causing irregularities, sharp folds, and other shape abnormalities |
| **Duration of results** | Permanent |

# CHEEK AUGMENTATION
*Malar augmentation*

## WHY HAVE CHEEK SURGERY?

High, prominent cheekbones are one of the facial features most associated with beauty and youth. Today, this underlying facial structure can be created with cheek augmentation surgery. Cheek augmentation changes the shape or size of the cheek and may correct flaws caused by birth defects or injury to give the face a more proportioned and balanced appearance. Cheek implants can give older patients with sunken or drawn cheeks a fuller look. Younger patients may choose cheek implant surgery to achieve a high-cheekboned look.

## What is the procedure?

Cheek augmentation involves the surgical insertion of cheek implants, or injections of fat or other dermal fillers. Cheek implants can be customized to fit each individual's face, and are made from several different types of materials including silicone and polyethylene. Rarely, various cuts to the zygomatic bone (cheekbone) may be performed. Cheek augmentation is also commonly combined with other procedures, such as facelift or chin augmentation. This procedure is generally performed on an outpatient basis, depending on whether other procedures are also being performed.

## Am I a candidate for cheek implant surgery?

**You may be a suitable candidate if you:**
- Are in good physical and emotional health
- Want to add definition to your face
- Have no allergies to the implant material
- Have realistic expectations for the outcome of your cheek implant surgery.

This is only a partial list of the criteria that your surgeon will consider in determining whether or not this procedure is appropriate for you. Certain medical conditions and medications may affect whether you are a suitable candidate for cheek augmentation surgery.

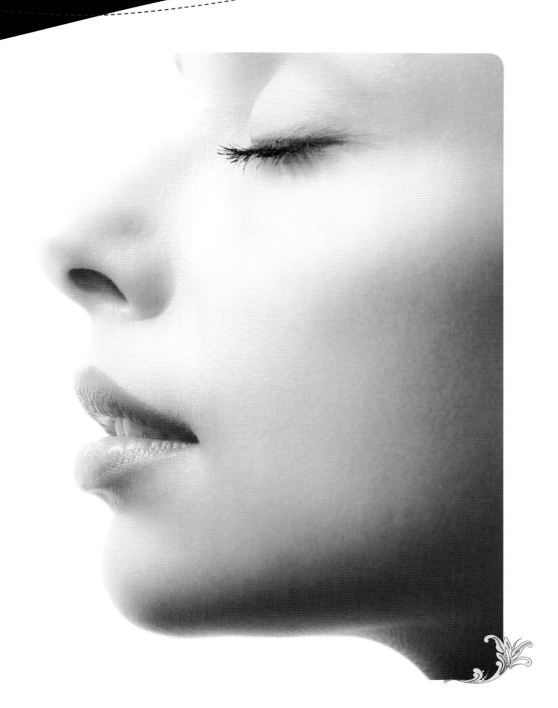

## The basic procedure

### 1. ANESTHESIA

You will be given general anesthesia, so you will be asleep during the operation.

### 2. THE INCISIONS

The surgeon makes two incisions inside the mouth between the upper gums and cheek, and then creates a small pocket over the cheekbones. The implant is inserted through the incisions and slid into place. A small titanium screw may be used to attach the cheek implant to the bone. When cheek implant

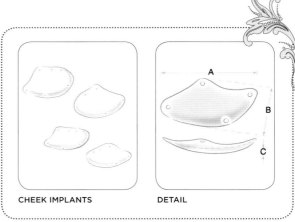

CHEEK IMPLANTS          DETAIL

**Cheek implant sizes vary depending on the volume required by the patient.**

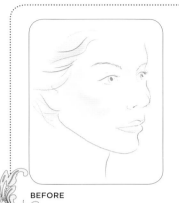
BEFORE

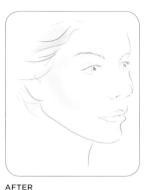
AFTER

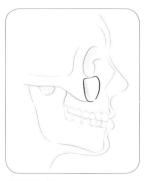
POSITION OF IMPLANT

surgery is performed with other facial procedures, the implants may be inserted through the incisions used for that procedure.

### 3. THE SUTURES
The incisions are sutured and a compression bandage applied.

### 4. THE RESULTS
Your face will be swollen immediately after the procedure. The end results of the cheek implant surgery may not be apparent for 3 or 4 months.

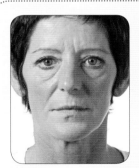

BEFORE

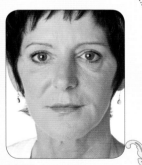
AFTER

**The result of the cheek implant surgery is a fresher, rejuvenated look.**

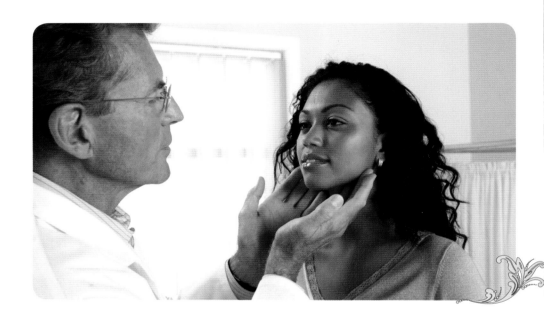

## Recovery and healing

You may experience some numbness, swelling, and bruising. Any pain can be controlled with medication. Keep your head elevated when resting or sleeping, and apply cold compresses to reduce swelling. Chewing, brushing teeth, smiling, and talking may be difficult for several days. Eat only soft foods and liquids.

Normal activities may be resumed in a few days and you may return to work after about 5 days. Avoid strenuous activity and rough contact near the face for at least 4 weeks.

Sutures are removed within a week, and absorbable sutures will dissolve in around 10 days. New facial contours emerge within 4–6 weeks, with the final results emerging about 7 months following cheek implant surgery.

# FACTS
## CHEEK AUGMENTATION

| | |
|---|---|
| **Description** | Insertion of cheek implants or fillers to create "cheekbones." |
| **Length of surgery** | 30–45 minutes |
| **In/outpatient** | Outpatient |
| **Anesthesia** | General |
| **Back to work in...** | 5 days |
| **Back to the gym in...** | 4 weeks |
| **Treatment frequency** | Once (or more with injectable fillers) |
| **Risks** | • Swelling<br>• Numbness<br>• Bruising<br>• Tightness in the cheeks<br>• Difficulty smiling, talking, and chewing<br>• Infection<br>• Bleeding<br>• Nerve damage<br>• Allergic reaction to the anesthetic<br>• Scarring<br>• The cheek implant may shift to another part of the face |
| **Duration of results** | Permanent (except for injectable fillers) |

# NECK LIFT
## *Platysmaplasty*

## *What is the procedure?*

The neck lift is a very popular procedure among women and men who have jowls or a "turkey wattle" appearance to the neck, often after excessive weight gain when the muscles and skin have been stretched. The neck can also age before your face, and if you've lost a lot of weight, your neck may retain loose or sagging skin. A neck lift is actually a pair of procedures used together to enhance the appearance of your neck:

- Cervicoplasty is the procedure used to remove excess skin

### WHY HAVE A NECK LIFT?

There are many different reasons why people choose to have a neck lift. The neck can age faster than the face and many patients only need a neck lift, rather than a full facelift. Aging does not always determine the need for a neck lift; often weight loss prompts it. Many patients choose to have a neck lift at the same time as their facelift procedure.

- Platysmaplasty removes or alters neck muscles.

## *Am I a candidate for a neck lift?*

For many people, the neck is the first place to show the signs of the aging process. If you have loose, hanging skin that has lost its elasticity, band lines, or excess skin or fat, a neck lift may help to bring your neck back into the tighter shape you desire.

### In general, the best candidates are:

- In good physical health
- Psychologically stable
- Wanting to improve their appearance
- Realistic in their expectations.

### WHAT TO EXPECT FROM A CONSULTATION WITH A NECK LIFT SURGEON

During the consultation the surgeon will discuss your reasons for wanting a neck lift, and your suitability for this type of procedure. Your age and medical history will be taken into account. You will be also be asked about your previous surgeries, past and present medical conditions, and treatments you have received, as well as any medications you are taking.

# The basic procedure

It is not uncommon for a cosmetic surgeon to perform neck liposuction during a neck lift, which removes excess fat. If you are having other surgeries in conjunction with a neck lift, such as liposuction, facelift, or brow lift, the duration of the surgery will be longer.

## 1. ANESTHESIA

The neck lift procedure starts with either a local or a general anesthetic.

## 2. THE INCISIONS

The incision sites for your neck lift will be marked. For a neck lift encompassing platysmaplasty (tightening of the neck muscles) with additional skin lift, a small incision is made under the chin and behind or under the ear to access the muscles in your neck. Some muscles may be manipulated or removed.

The skin can be brought together under or behind the ear to further firm up the appearance of the neck. Cervicoplasty surgery corrects loose and sagging skin. The surgeon will make similar incisions, trim the skin, move it into place, and secure it with stitches or tissue glue. Surgeons may use endoscopic or "keyhole" techniques.

## 3. THE SUTURES

The neck lift incisions are normally closed with either non-dissolvable or dissolvable sutures or tissue glue. Those around your hairline will be closed with small metal staples. You will have a pressure dressing placed around

**Swelling normally subsides 3 to 5 days following neck lift surgery.**

your head, wrapped around from the top, covering your ears, and under your chin. It is possible that your surgeon may place a drain under the skin on the neck to collect any fluid that may cause discomfort.

## 4. THE RESULTS

After surgery you will be taken to the recovery room; your neck may feel tight and quite tender as the anesthesia wears off. You may feel a little nauseous as a result of the anesthesia. You may also feel some pain, but your neck lift surgeon will prescribe you medication to relieve this. Your neck will be very swollen for about 3 days, and there will be some bruising and numbness. After the swelling has eased, the neck should appear firmer, less lined, and more "youthful" in appearance.

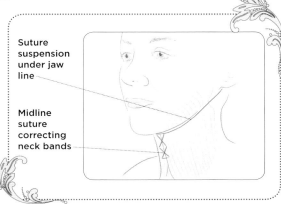

Suture suspension under jaw line

Midline suture correcting neck bands

## Preparing for neck lift surgery

The first thing you should do to prepare for neck lift surgery is talk to your surgeon and inform him or her about any pre-existing medical conditions and any medications you are taking, and follow any pre-operation directions you are given. You will probably be advised to stop smoking a few weeks before the surgery to speed up the post-operative healing process. Most people are also advised to eat healthily, because the body will need nutrients to heal.

## Recovery and healing

Make sure that you have arranged for someone to drive you home after surgery, and that there will be someone with you for the first 24 hours in case of complications.

You may need to wear a compression bandage for 1 week after surgery and the neck may be swollen and bruised for a number of days. Sleep in an elevated position for 2 weeks to help the swelling subside. There may be some numbness or pain, replaced by itching or a burning sensation, which can take up to 6 months to stop as the nerves heal.

You may have drainage tubes in place, which can be removed after 1–2 days, and any remaining stitches can be removed after 10 days. When you leave the hospital, 1–2 days after your neck lift procedure, you will need to take 1–2 weeks off work and avoid any strenuous activity for 2–3 weeks. Avoid contact sports for 6–8 weeks.

## Tips for a speedy recovery:

- Get as much rest as possible— give yourself time to heal
- If you are in pain, take your prescribed painkillers
- Take your temperature regularly— an elevated temperature could signify an infection
- Don't bend over or lift heavy objects for 3 weeks
- Avoid alcohol and aspirin
- If you are a smoker and have stopped for the procedure, don't start again!

## FACTS
### NECK LIFT SURGERY

| | |
|---|---|
| **Description** | A pair of procedures used together to enhance the appearance of your neck. |
| **Length of surgery** | 2–3 hours |
| **In/outpatient** | Inpatient or outpatient |
| **Anesthesia** | Local or general |
| **Back to work in...** | 1–2 weeks |
| **Back to the gym in...** | 2–3 weeks |
| **Treatment frequency** | One or more times as desired |
| **Risks** | • Swelling<br>• Bruising<br>• Numbness<br>• A tingling or burning sensation<br>• Skin tightness or pulling<br>• Infection<br>• Allergic reaction to the anesthetic<br>• Problems with wound healing<br>• Bleeding under the skin (hematoma)<br>• Fluid buildup under the skin (seroma)<br>• Permanent scarring in the neck area with red and unsightly scars<br>• Permanent nerve damage<br>• Asymmetry<br>• Lumpiness and/or mottling of the skin<br>• Laxity relapse of the muscles and skin of the neck<br>• Dissatisfaction with the results |
| **Duration of results** | 5–10 years |

# BROW LIFT
## *Forehead lift*

### WHY HAVE A BROW LIFT?

Brow lift or forehead lift surgery can make you look younger and fresher by improving the appearance of your face. The results of a brow lift procedure will be good if you have good skin tone, your skin has not lost its elasticity, and moves and stretches easily. Your face is made up of layers of bone, muscle, fascia, fat, and skin. During the natural aging process, the muscles lose their tone, and the fascia slackens.

## *What is the procedure?*

A brow lift is often performed to treat conditions associated with aging, commonly on patients between 40 and 60 years of age. However, the procedure can also be carried out on younger adults who have developed furrows or frown lines due to stress, muscle activity, or inherited conditions, such as a low, heavy brow or furrowed lines above the nose.

A brow lift may be performed in conjunction with other cosmetic procedures to achieve a more harmonious facial appearance.

## *Am I a candidate for brow lift surgery?*

If you are concerned by any of the following, you could benefit:

- Sagging brow
- Forehead wrinkling
- Deep creases between the eyebrows and on the bridge of the nose
- Deep furrows between the eyes.

### WHAT TO EXPECT FROM A CONSULTATION WITH A BROW LIFT SURGEON

The consultation will typically include a discussion of your individual objectives, the options available for a brow lift/facial rejuvenation, the likely outcome of the surgical procedure, and details of any risks or complications associated with the operation.

The surgeon will also evaluate your overall health. The success and overall safety of a brow lift procedure (as with any other surgery) requires that you are realistic about your expectations, and are honest about your medical history and use of medications, herbal supplements, alcohol, drugs, and tobacco.

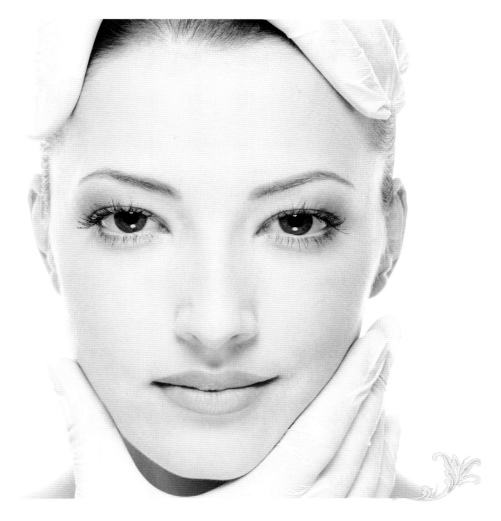

## A BROW LIFT CAN:

- Reduce furrows and other signs of aging in the forehead and brow areas, creating a softer, rejuvenated appearance
- Minimize the creases and lines that develop across the forehead and high on the bridge of the nose
- Improve frown lines that appear as vertical creases between the eyebrows
- Reposition low or sagging brows that may hood the upper eyelids
- Raise eyebrows to a more fresh, alert, and youthful position.

# The basic procedure

A brow lift is often performed in conjunction with a facelift or eyelid surgery. The procedure can be performed by making a long incision either in front of or behind the hairline, above the ears. The incision is designed to be inconspicuous once healed.

Through the incision, the surgeon can modify or remove parts of the muscles that cause wrinkling and frown lines, remove excess skin, and lift your eyebrows to a more aesthetically pleasing level. The skin and deeper layers are then fixed to the bone. The soft tissues of the forehead are tightened to restore a more youthful contour to the upper face. This is called a coronal brow lift. Occasionally, incisions may be performed in the forehead, and/or the upper eyelids.

Another type of brow lift procedure uses an endoscope—a long, thin tube with a light on the end—attached to a video camera. The endoscope is inserted through 4-6 tiny incisions in the scalp and through these incisions the surgeon can work on the internal structures of the forehead. The endoscopic technique has the advantage of requiring very minimal incisions, but it may not be possible for all patients. Some brow lift patients may benefit from a combination of endoscopic and other techniques.

If your main concern is frown lines between your eyebrows or across the top of your nose, a limited endoscopic brow lift to correct these problems can be performed.

## 1. ANESTHESIA

The anesthetic choices for brow lift surgery include intravenous sedation and general anesthetic. Your surgeon will recommend the best choice for you. You will be given a relaxant in the form of a tablet, followed by an injection containing an antibiotic and an anesthetic, and then finally a local anesthetic.

## 2. THE INCISIONS

**Endoscopic brow lift**—Four to six small incisions are made within the hairline and an endoscope with a light and camera on the end and special instruments are inserted through these cuts. This allows the brow lift surgeon to reposition, alter, or remove the tissue and muscle beneath the skin to correct the source of visible creases and furrows in the forehead.

Correction of a low-positioned or sagging brow may be made with or without the use of an endoscope through incisions at the temples and in the scalp. This technique may be done in conjunction with incisions hidden within the natural crease of the upper eyelids to eliminate frown lines between the brows, and on or above the bridge of the nose.

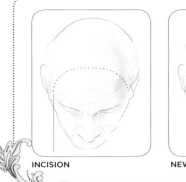

INCISION

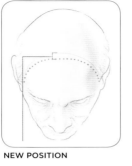

NEW POSITION

**Left and below: Incisions are made to the top of the head or from behind the hairline from ear to ear.**

**Coronal brow lift**—The incision is made across the top of your head or behind the hairline, from ear to ear. Through this incision, your surgeon can alter the muscles that cause horizontal forehead wrinkles and scowling. The surgeon will remove a $1/2$–1 inch (1–2 cm) strip of scalp and sew the remaining scalp together. The advantage of this technique is that it is lasting (it will not have to be repeated as you age, with very rare exceptions). Also, the scars are concealed behind the hairline. Recovery time is often longer than the endoscopic brow lift due to the size of the incision.

## 3. CLOSING THE INCISIONS
Brow lift incisions are typically closed with removable or absorbable sutures, skin adhesives, surgical tape, and/or special clips.

## 4. THE RESULTS
A bandage may be wrapped around your forehead or face. Any discomfort you feel will be controlled with pain medication. You may be permitted to go home after a few hours, although some patients may stay overnight. The results will appear gradually as the swelling and bruising subside to reveal smoother forehead skin and a more youthful, rested appearance. The effects can be maintained by the use of permanent sutures, small surgical screws, or an absorbable fixation device at the temples.

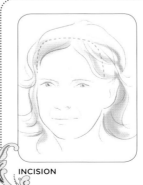

INCISION

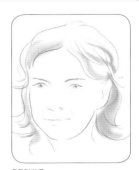

RESULT

# Recovery and healing

Recovery times vary from patient to patient and smokers take longer to heal. You may need pain relief to help with any discomfort as the anesthetic wears off. Your surgeon will prescribe painkillers.

You will need to arrange for someone to drive you home. You should try to have a friend or relative stay with you for the first 24 hours. Your nurse will give you some advice about caring for your healing wounds and a date for a follow-up appointment.

You will experience some swelling and bruising in the 10–14 day period following brow lift surgery. In some patients, this condition may include the cheek and eye area as well as the forehead. You may develop black eyes temporarily.

Keeping your head elevated, including sleeping propped up on pillows, and using cold compresses will help to reduce swelling.

As the incisions heal, you may experience some numbness and itching, but these will subside with time. The sutures are usually removed within 7 to 10 days following surgery, or will dissolve on their own. If bandages have been used, they are removed in 1–3 days.

For most patients, the recovery time will not exceed 2 weeks, but patients may still be advised to avoid strenuous activities for longer periods. Rest as much as possible in the first week following surgery, and keep your incision sites as dry as possible.

Healing will continue for several weeks as the swelling dissipates and incision lines refine and fade and it may take several months for you to completely recover and see the final results of your brow lift.

# Preparing for brow lift surgery

Your surgeon will explain the procedure you will undergo. Prior to surgery you will be given instructions to help you prepare for surgery, which may include:

- Pre-surgical lab tests or diagnostic testing
- Day-of-surgery instructions and medications
- Instructions regarding the use of anesthesia
- Post-operative care and follow-up instructions.

# FACTS
## BROW LIFT SURGERY

| | |
|---|---|
| **Description** | Surgery to improve the appearance of the face by removing furrows. |
| **Length of surgery** | 30–90 minutes |
| **In/outpatient** | Inpatient or outpatient |
| **Anesthesia** | General or intravenous sedation |
| **Back to work in...** | 1–2 weeks |
| **Back to the gym in...** | 3–4 weeks |
| **Treatment frequency** | One or more times as desired |
| **Risks** | • Soreness, swelling, and bruising—this can last up to a month<br>• Scarring—this usually fades over the course of a year, but won't completely disappear<br>• Raised hairline in front of, and behind, your ears<br>• Unfavorable scarring<br>• Nerve damage—injury to the nerves that control movement of the eyebrows<br>• Loss of sensation—this numbness is usually temporary, but it can be permanent<br>• Hematoma<br>• Infection<br>• Poor wound healing<br>• Skin loss<br>• Seroma<br>• Skin contour irregularities<br>• Skin discoloration, sensitivity, and swelling<br>• Deep vein thrombosis<br>• Dissatisfaction with results |
| **Duration of results** | 5–10 years |

# LIP AUGMENTATION
## Lip implants

### WHY HAVE LIP AUGMENTATION?

Lip-augmentation procedures enhance the fullness of lips. Like the rest of our skin, our lips lose collagen and fat during the aging process. Other factors that accelerate the signs of aging include smoking and sun exposure. Lip augmentation is ideal for patients who have always had naturally thin lips, and also for those who want to return their lips to the shape and fullness they had when they were younger. This is accomplished by implanting synthetic or biological materials into the lips to make them plumper and more appealing.

## What is the procedure?

Most people who are thinking about lip enhancement want fuller lips that are smooth, plump, wrinkle-free, and youthful-looking.

If you are interested in lip augmentation, you have a variety of options. There are several techniques used in lip enhancement; some are more invasive than others. The two main options are surgery and injections of various types of filler materials. The results of such lip injections generally do not last, as most of them are broken down in the body within several months and must be repeated on a regular basis for most people.

## Am I a candidate for lip augmentation?

**Reasons for lip enhancement include:**
- Desiring a sensuous, plump look for your lips
- "Balancing" the facial features
- Restoring lost volume and shape
- Increasing self-confidence.

**WHAT TO EXPECT FROM A CONSULTATION WITH A LIP AUGMENTATION SURGEON**
You will discuss options for your lip augmentation, anesthesia, incision placements, and risks. If you are getting an injection you will require an allergy test, and you may have it during this meeting. In this case you would have a little bit of the substance to be used injected into the crook of your arm and be instructed to watch the injection site closely for several weeks. You would need to report any signs of inflammation to your surgeon.

# The basic procedure

Traditional lip implants usually last at least 2 years but, as the mouth area moves so much, there is a risk that they may shift to other parts of the face.

Fat-injection lip enhancement is the next longest-lasting technique; how long these implants last is dependent on the length of time it takes for the fat to be absorbed back into the individual's body.

The safest option for lip augmentation is generally considered to be collagen lip injections, though repeat treatment will be needed about every 9–12 weeks. The collagen lip injection procedure has been proven to be a safe and effective treatment, and these injections are becoming increasingly popular, though there is a small risk of allergy.

Although you may favor the injections over the surgical option, bear in mind that lip augmentation surgery may be less expensive in the long run when you consider the number of repeat injections you would need.

## SURGERY

Lip augmentation surgery involves inserting implants into the lips to achieve a fuller appearance. There are several different substances commonly used in lip augmentation procedures, each with their own particular features and techniques:

- **AlloDerm:** The most popular material for lip augmentation. It is a natural collagen sheet harvested from cadavers and is screened and highly processed within very strict standards.

The risk of infection is approximately 2 percent. The patient has a local anesthetic, the material is inserted through tiny incisions made in the inside corners of the mouth, then stitches are used to close the incisions. AlloDerm eventually integrates with the natural tissues of the body. The material can be absorbed, so the results are only temporary, lasting from 6 months to 1 year.

- **Synthetic implants:** Gore-Tex®, SoftForm™, and soft ePTFE are other synthetic options with permanent results. They do not shrink, cannot be absorbed into the body, and remain in place because scar tissue forms on either end.

The implants are inserted by making a small incision in the inside of the lip. The material is then made into the shape of a small tube and inserted with a small needle. Synthetic implants are foreign bodies and may become infected or be rejected by the body. They can, however, also be removed.

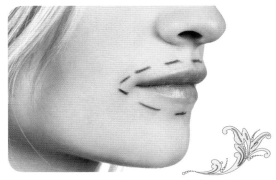

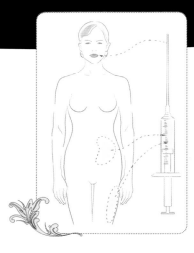

**Fat can be removed from another area of the body and injected into the lips.**

- **Fat grafting:** Many people choose fat grafting (see above) because they are comfortable with the idea of using fat from their own body. The fat is harvested from another area of the body, often the abdomen or thighs. It is prepared and inserted with a needle into the lip from more than one point. This procedure has permanent results in approximately half who try it, although the body may reabsorb the implants.
- **Local flap grafts**: Local flaps bring material from inside the mouth to enhance the lips on the outside. An incision may be made inside the mouth to push the tissue inside the mouth upward and outward into the lip, sometimes in conjunction with grafting. Alternatively, an incision may be made along the upper lip line. In this case, skin above the lip is removed, and the lip is then stitched along the line of the incision. The results are temporary.

## INJECTIONS

Lip injection procedures are performed as an outpatient procedure, and patients usually return to normal activities within 2–3 days. The main drawback of lip enhancement injections is that the fat or collagen is absorbed back into the body over time and repeat treatments are required to maintain the result. It can be a good way, however, to see what fuller lips could look like on you before you consider a more permanent procedure. The following are some of the lip injection options available:

- **Collagen injections:** Prepared from the collagen found in cow skin, collagen injections are used to temporarily augment the lips. Collagen may cause allergic reactions in some people, therefore a sensitivity test should be performed before the lip augmentation procedure goes ahead. The body eventually absorbs the collagen; results last between 1 and 3 months.
- **Fat injections:** Fat is harvested from another area of the body (often the abdomen or thighs), purified, and injected into the lips. There is no possibility of allergic reaction. Results usually last longer than collagen. However, lumping or scarring may result.
- **ArteColl injections:** ArteColl is composed mainly of tiny synthetic beads (polymethyl methacrylate)

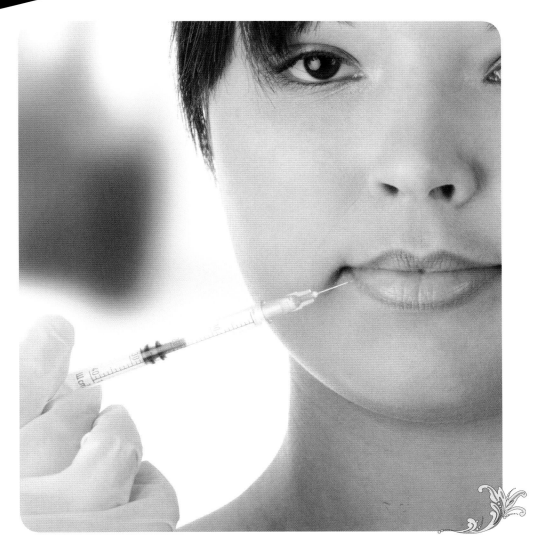

injected into the lips to raise them. Lasts longer than fat or collagen.

- **Autologen injections:** Autologen is collagen extracted from the patient's own skin; often from excess skin removed in a facelift. The results are relatively long-lasting.

- **Restylane injections:** Restylane is a clear gel, a component of which is similar to one naturally found in the body.

The material in the following injections is harvested from human tissue:

- **Dermalogen injections:** Dermalogen is extracted from the skin of a cadaver, screened, and processed to avoid the spread of disease. The effects are temporary.
- **Fascia injections:** Fascia (white connective tissue) extracted from a cadaver may be injected or surgically implanted.

- **HylaForm injections:** Tissue extracted from a cadaver, screened, and processed, is injected into the lips. It is gradually absorbed into the body over 6–12 months.

For most types of lip enhancement, the treatment must be repeated on a regular basis for the best results. Make sure that you discuss your expectations fully with the surgeon before you undergo any procedure.

## Recovery and healing

After the procedure, you may experience some pain and swelling. This usually lasts a few days, and your recovery will depend on which type of lip enhancement you underwent. If you had injections, recovery may take just two days, though the swelling or bruising may last longer. If you had implants or grafts, recovery may take up to two weeks.

**Tips for a speedy recovery:**
- Apply ice packs to your lips intermittently for the first 48 hours
- Take painkillers if you need them
- Take antiobiotics if prescribed
- Drink lots of fluids

- Take your temperature regularly— an elevated temperature over 101°F (38°C) can indicate an infection
- Don't take any aspirin or drink alcohol for at least 2 weeks
- Limit talking and chewing during the first 48 hours
- Limit smiling and laughing for the first week (if you can!)
- Sleep in a semi-upright position for the first week
- Don't bend over, strain, exercise, or take part in any activities that could increase pressure on your lips
- Avoid strenuous activities for 1–3 days
- Keep the lips clean.

# FACTS
## LIP AUGMENTATION SURGERY

| | |
|---|---|
| **Description** | Lip augmentation procedures enhance the fullness of lips and make them more attractive. |
| **Length of surgery** | Up to 2 hours (depending on procedure) |
| **In/outpatient** | Outpatient |
| **Anesthesia** | Local or topical (depending on procedure) |
| **Back to work in...** | 2–3 days |
| **Back to the gym in...** | 2–3 days |
| **Treatment frequency** | Some need repeating every few months; depends on procedure |
| **Risks** | • Swelling<br>• Bruising<br>• Redness or bleeding around the lip outline<br>• Cold sores<br>• Numbness<br>• Hard spots if the artificial collagen did not set properly in the tissues<br>• Asymmetrical lips<br>• Loss of natural lip line<br>• Permanent stiffness in the lip<br>• Implant material may move to a new location within the lips and/or protrude unnaturally<br>• Allergic reactions<br>• Fat injections can cause lumping or scarring<br>• Implant made from foreign substances may become infected or be rejected by the body |
| **Duration of results** | Varies |

# NOSE SURGERY
## *Rhinoplasty*

## *What is the procedure?*

During a rhinoplasty, the nasal cartilage and bones are modified to make the nose smaller (reduction rhinoplasty), or tissue is added (augmentation rhinoplasty). The change can be made by adding or removing bone or cartilage, grafting tissue from another part of the body, or implanting synthetic material to alter the shape of the nose. Aesthetic improvements also include altering the tip or bridge of the nose, and narrowing or changing the shape of the nostrils. Nose surgery is also frequently performed to repair nasal fractures, or if a patient has breathing difficulties.

## WHY HAVE NOSE SURGERY?

Nose surgery, or rhinoplasty, (commonly referred to as a "nose job") is a cosmetic procedure, usually performed to enhance the appearance of the nose. The term "rhinoplasty" literally means "nose molding" or "nose forming." Rhinoplasty is a very popular procedure that can make profound differences not only to the symmetry, shape, and size of facial features, but also to a person's self-esteem.

## *Am I a candidate for rhinoplasty?*

Before you decide to undergo rhinoplasty, you should be certain that it is really what you want. Your nose is the most prominent feature on your face, and changing its shape can drastically alter your appearance. It is essential that you have realistic expectations.

Discussing your expectations with your surgeon is very important, to ensure that your goals are compatible with what is surgically possible. Nose surgery candidates should be at least in their mid teens, so that the nasal bone has matured and the shape of the nose has stabilized.

**You may be a good candidate for rhinoplasty surgery if:**
- Your facial growth is complete and you are 13 years of age or older
- You are physically and mentally healthy
- You have specific and, importantly, realistic goals for the results of your nose surgery.

**A good candidate for nose-reshaping:**

- Has a nose that he or she feels is too large or too small in comparison to other facial features
- Has a bump on the bridge of the nose
- Has a wide nose
- Has a nasal tip that droops, protrudes, or is enlarged
- Has a bulbous nose tip
- Has nostrils that are excessively flared or pinched
- Has a nose that is crooked or off-center
- Has been injured so that the nose is asymmetrical
- Has problems breathing due to irregularities with the internal nose structure.

## WHAT TO EXPECT FROM A CONSULTATION WITH A RHINOPLASTY SURGEON

During your consultation you will have the opportunity to discuss all aspects of the procedure at length. The surgeon will first discuss what you want to achieve, then use his expertise to assess your motivation for undergoing the procedure. The surgeon will also ask questions about your medical history to ensure there are no existing conditions that could make surgery risky or unfeasible. You will be advised of your options for surgery, and which is the best choice for you, and whether general anesthetic or IV sedation is required.

## Preparing for rhinoplasty

Before you set foot in the operating room, you can begin preparing for your surgery. The steps you take will help to ensure the safety and success of your procedure and ease recovery. Your surgeon will give you specific preparatory instructions, which may include the following:

- You must be free from any respiratory infections, coughs, and colds
- Smokers will be asked to stop smoking, because it increases the risk of infection

- The operation is conducted under general anesthetic, so you will be required to abstain from eating and drinking for about 6 hours before anesthesia is administered
- Avoid taking anti-inflammatory medications or herbal supplements because they can increase the risk of bleeding
- If you are currently taking medications, you may be advised to stop these or adjust the schedule.

# The basic procedure

## 1. ANESTHESIA

Depending on the extent of the procedure that you are undergoing, you will either receive intravenous sedation or general anesthetic. Your doctor will recommend the best choice for you, taking your individual factors into account.

## 2. THE INCISIONS AND RE-SHAPING OF THE NOSE

**Closed procedure:** Small incisions are made inside the nose to reach the bone and cartilage. Some is removed or rearranged to achieve the shape you have agreed with your surgeon. The skin over your nose is left untouched and shrinks to the new shape.

**Open procedure:** An incision is made across the columella, the narrow strip of tissue that separates the nostrils. The soft tissues that cover the nose are gently raised, allowing the surgeon access to reshape the structure of the nose.

To keep your features in proportion, it may be necessary to make your nostrils smaller. This is done by making cuts in the skin of the nostrils, which will leave fine scars on each side of your nostrils.

If you are having augmentation rhinoplasty, you may need a graft of extra bone or cartilage to build up your nose. Most commonly, pieces of cartilage from the septum, the partition in the middle of the nose, are used for this purpose. Cartilage may also be taken from your ears, or bone may be taken from your elbow, a rib, the skull, or the hip. Sometimes artificial implants are used instead.

## 3. CLOSING THE INCISIONS

Once the underlying structure of the nose is sculpted to the desired shape, the nasal skin and tissue is redraped and the cuts are closed with dissolvable stitches. You may also have small plastic splints inserted inside your nose to prevent scar tissue from

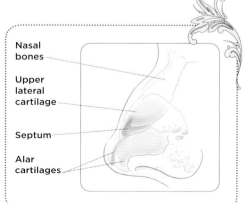

Nasal bones

Upper lateral cartilage

Septum

Alar cartilages

**Left: Nasal surgery is commonly performed to correct nasal fractures and breathing difficulties.**

forming and support the nose as it begins to heal.

## 4. THE RESULTS

The initial swelling will subside within a few weeks, and you may notice gradual changes in the appearance of your nose as it refines to a more permanent outcome. This takes around a year.

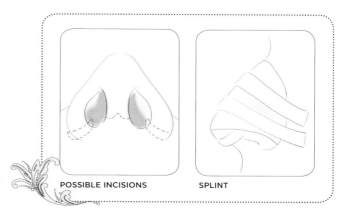

POSSIBLE INCISIONS          SPLINT

## *Recovery and healing*

When you come round from the procedure, you will have packs (dressings) in each nostril for about a day, which will stop you from breathing through your nose. You may be asked to stay in hospital overnight, so that the packs can be removed in the morning. You will also have a splint over your nose to support it for 7–10 days. Dissolvable stitches will disappear on their own in 7–10 days.

Rest until the effects of the anesthetic have subsided, and take any pain medication prescribed to you to help relieve any discomfort as the anesthetic wears off.

Ensure that you arrange for someone to drive you home, and have a friend or relative stay with you for the first 24 hours. When you go home, you can take over-the-counter painkillers such as paracetamol or ibuprofen. You may

experience some minor nosebleeds for a few days. It will take several months before your nose settles into its new shape.

### Tips for a speedy recovery:

- Keep your head up as much as possible to reduce the risk of bleeding
- Don't have a hot bath or drink alcohol for 2 weeks
- Don't use any nasal sprays or decongestants. Sleeping propped up on several pillows will help to relieve congestion
- You will need to breathe through your mouth for the first few days, which can lead to dry lips. Use lip balm to soothe cracked lips
- Don't blow your nose for at least a week. If you need to sneeze, cough it out.

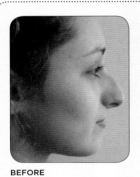

BEFORE

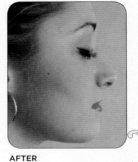

AFTER

**Rhinoplasty can give a symmetrical, balanced look to the facial profile.**

## FACTS
### NOSE SURGERY

| | |
|---|---|
| Description | Cosmetic procedure performed to enhance the appearance of the nose. |
| Length of surgery | 1–2 hours |
| In/Outpatient | Outpatient |
| Anesthesia | General |
| Back to work in... | 7–10 days |
| Back to the gym in... | 2 weeks |
| Treatment frequency | Once |

# FACTS
## NOSE SURGERY

**Risks**

- Soreness, swelling, and bruising, particularly around your eyes—this can last up to a month
- Stiffness and numbness, particularly at the nose tip—numbness can last a few months but stiffness may be permanent
- Inability to breathe through the nose—this should ease as the swelling settles
- Scarring—though you should have little or no scarring on your nose, you will have permanent scars on your hip or chest if you have had bone taken from there
- Red spots on your skin's surface caused by burst small blood vessels—may be temporary or permanent
- Scarring—the scars won't be visible, but you may be able to feel them for a while after surgery
- Open-nose surgery procedure may give you a small scar on the underside of the nose
- Revision rhinoplasty—in around one case in 10, the patient needs to have additional minor surgery to correct a slight deformity
- Chest or nose infection—treatable with antibiotics
- Heavy nosebleed either shortly after the operation, or after a week to 10 days
- Temporary loss of or reduction in sensitivity to smell—this may be permanent
- Changes in the shape of the nose as scar tissue matures
- Damage to the septum
- If you've had an implant, it's possible it may push through the lining of your nose and need to be removed

**Duration of results**

Permanent

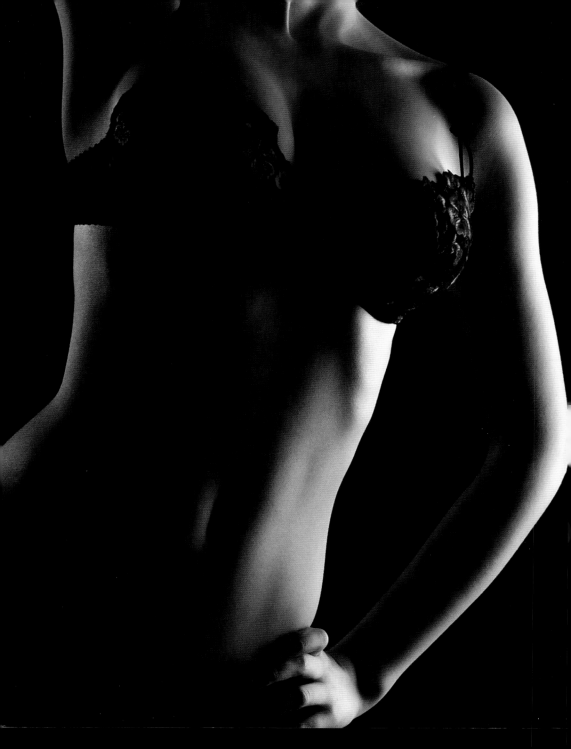

# CHAPTER THREE
# BREAST COSMETIC SURGERY

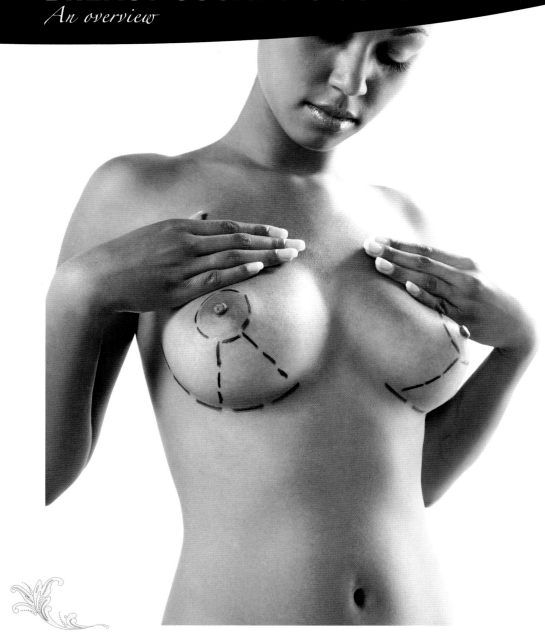

Breast surgery is one of the most popular areas of cosmetic surgery and includes several procedures. Breast augmentation (enlargement) is usually accomplished with breast implants. Breast lift (mastopexy) is a procedure that is often performed at the same time as augmentation. In addition to these purely cosmetic procedures, breast reduction (reduction mammoplasty) is an enhancement surgery that potentially offers both cosmetic and health benefits, while breast reconstruction is a procedure often performed following a mastectomy (removal of the breast).

Whether your breasts are too large, too small, or not as firm or as shapely as you would like, surgery is one way to help make you feel more confident and feminine again. Women often seek cosmetic breast surgery if they have:

- Small breasts
- Asymmetrical breasts
- Suffered from breast cancer and have had a mastectomy
- Reduced firmness due to aging
- Drooping or sagging breasts after child bearing and breastfeeding.

The most important step is to locate a reputable, board-certified cosmetic surgeon, and organize a consultation to find out more about what the surgery entails and how it may meet your requirements. The surgeon will explain the options available to you, including the different types of procedures; this information should also include the risks, side effects, and limitations, as well as the costs and likely outcomes.

*A good candidate for breast surgery is:*

- 18 years of age or older
- Not currently pregnant or nursing
- In good physical health
- Psychologically stable
- Wanting to improve their appearance
- Realistic in their expectations
- Having this surgery for the first time.

## BREAST AUGMENTATION

A breast augmentation, or enlargement, is surgery to increase the size of the breasts or correct asymmetrical breasts. It usually involves placing an implant under either the breast tissue or the chest muscle behind the breast. You may choose to enlarge your breasts if you feel that they are too small, or perhaps you want to increase their size after losing weight or following a pregnancy, or you want to correct a difference in size between the two breasts. The operation may also be offered if you are having reconstructive surgery as part of treatment for breast cancer or other conditions that may affect the size and shape of your breasts.

## BREAST RECONSTRUCTION

Breast reconstruction is an operation to try to get back the shape of the breast after mastectomy (removal of a breast), or lumpectomy (removal of part of the breast). The aim of a breast reconstruction is to match the remaining natural breast as closely as possible. This can either be done by creating a breast "form" with a breast implant, or by using natural tissue from another part of your body. If you have lost one or both breasts, the creation of a new breast can dramatically improve your self-image, self-confidence, and quality of life. However, although breast reconstruction surgery can give you a relatively natural-looking breast, a reconstructed breast will never look or feel exactly the same as the breast that was removed. Breast reconstruction typically involves several procedures performed in multiple stages. It can begin at the same time as the mastectomy, or you can delay it until you heal from the mastectomy and recover from any additional cancer treatments.

## BREAST REDUCTION

Breast reduction (or reduction mammoplasty) is a cosmetic surgery procedure that lifts the breast and makes it smaller. Women with large breasts often suffer from back pain, neck pain, breast pain, and other medical problems, and reduction surgery will help to relieve the symptoms. For this reason, it is considered a reconstructive surgery and is often covered by insurance. During the breast reduction, excess tissue and skin are removed from the breasts. The breasts are then reshaped to form smaller ones, and the nipples are repositioned. Breast asymmetry is common and liposuction of the breast can be a useful aletrnative to the other surgical options in some cases.

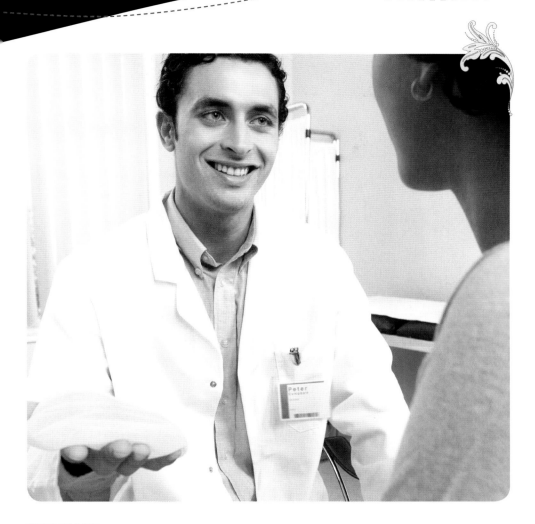

## BREAST LIFT

Breast lift (mastopexy) is an operation to raise and reshape your breasts if they have lost their shape and skin elasticity through pregnancy, breastfeeding, a loss or gain in weight, or as part of the aging process. There are several different techniques, depending on the degree of sagging. Breast lift surgery consists of removing excess skin from around the areola to tighten the skin that surrounds the breast. By tightening the skin in this way, the breast is "lifted," elevating the position of the nipple and areola. Some women may choose to have breast implants inserted in conjunction with a breast lift, which may yield more satisfying results for those who desire greater volume as well as firmness in their breasts.

# BREAST ENLARGEMENT
*Breast augmentation*

Most people choosing to have breast enlargement want to improve their self-esteem and self-image, and a breast augmentation procedure can help to improve their appearance and increase their self-confidence. Women who have suffered breast cancer can use breast implants for reconstructive purposes after mastectomy, or women with asymmetrical breasts may use a single breast implant to balance the difference in size. Following pregnancy, many women opt for breast implants to correct reductions in breast size.

## What is a breast augmentation?

Breast implants are available in a variety of shapes and sizes. An implant can be made of natural body tissue or synthetic material, such as silicone (a cohesive gel) or saline (salt water). Natural-tissue implants are usually only used on women having breast reconstruction surgery and are rarely used for cosmetic purposes.

Breast implants generally do not last a lifetime. If you decide to have a breast enlargement, you should take into account the possible future financial cost of further breast implant surgery (breast revision).

## Am I a candidate for breast augmentation surgery?

Undergoing a breast augmentation operation is a personal decision, but you may benefit from talking to your family and friends about it, or even someone who has had a breast augmentation procedure themselves. It is unwise to have breast implants to please someone else, and you should be sure that your decision is based upon your own needs.

You may be a suitable candidate if:
- Your breasts are uneven in size
- You feel that your breasts are too small
- Your breasts have lost the shape and size that you desire following dramatic weight loss or childbirth
- You have a congenital deformity
- You want to improve the way you feel and appear in your clothes.

Your age and health are also important determining factors. If you have malignant, or pre-malignant breast cancer that has not been treated, or if you have an infection, then the procedure is not suitable for you.

## WHAT TO EXPECT FROM A CONSULTATION WITH A BREAST AUGMENTATION SURGEON

This will include discussion about the type of breast implant that is most appropriate for you. There are many shapes, sizes, and materials from which to choose. Your surgeon will recommend the best for you.

One of the things you will want to know from the surgeon is how many breast implant surgeries they perform each year. You may also want to ask to speak with other patients who have undergone breast augmentation surgery there, and ask to see their book of before and after photos to assess the results of their work.

You may have a medical examination, during which the surgeon and a nurse will examine your breasts. The surgeon will assess the position of your nipples and the crease under each breast. They will also assess the symmetry of your breasts and nipples; their size, shape, and position. The examination may involve a light prodding and poking, so be prepared. The surgeon will also be testing the elasticity of you skin.

After the consultation with the doctor you will have about 20 minutes to try on a variety of different breast implant silicone sizers with one of the nurses. The sizer is placed inside a bra, often a sports bra, which you put on and can assess in front of a mirror to judge how you might look after the surgery.

## Preparing for breast augmentation surgery

If you smoke, you will be asked to stop in advance of the breast enlargement procedure. Aspirin and certain anti-inflammatory drugs can cause increased bleeding, so you should avoid taking these medications for a period of time before surgery. Your surgeon may also recommend a baseline mammogram before surgery and another mammographic examination some months afterward.

The procedure is usually carried out under a general anesthetic. You will not be able to eat or drink for about 6 hours beforehand; some anesthetists allow occasional sips of water.

Bring in a soft, supportive bra without underwiring to wear after surgery. Your surgeon will advise you about the most suitable type.

The surgeon will measure your breasts, assess their shape and the position of your nipples, and may mark the position of the incisions. With your consent, photographs may be taken, so that the results of your breast enlargement can be compared with your original appearance

# The basic procedure

## 1. ANESTHETIC

Breast implant operations are usually carried out under general anesthetic, though sometimes your surgeon will use intravenous sedation. It is possible to have a breast augmentation operation as day surgery, though you will normally need to stay in hospital overnight. The length of the procedure varies according to the technique used, the placement of the implants, the patient's anatomy, and the type of anesthesia.

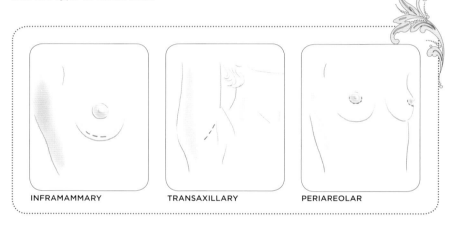

INFRAMAMMARY          TRANSAXILLARY          PERIAREOLAR

## 2. THE INCISIONS

Your surgeon will first make an incision, or cut, in an inconspicuous area to minimize visible scarring. You will be able to discuss these options with your surgeon before the operation to decide on the one that is best for you. Incisions vary based on the type of breast implant, degree of enlargement desired, your anatomy, and where you would like the scars to be.

Incision options include:

- **Inframammary**—a small cut is made in the fold beneath each breast.
- **Transaxillary**—a cut is made in your armpit, and may cause more visible scarring than the other two types.
- **Periareolar**—this incision, made around the nipple, causes only minimal scarring, though there is a possibility that nipple sensation may be affected.

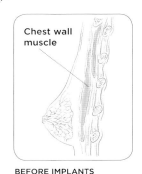

**Chest wall muscle**

BEFORE IMPLANTS

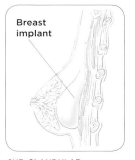

**Breast implant**

SUB-GLANDULAR PLACEMENT

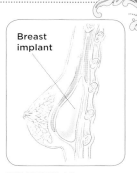

**Breast implant**

SUB-MUSCULAR PLACEMENT

- **Transumbilical**—saline breast implants are fitted by first going through an incision in the belly button area with a thin instrument.

After the incision has been made, the implant is inserted either beneath the breast tissue (sub-mammary/sub-glandular) or under the pectoral muscle (sub-muscular). Again, your surgeon will advise you on the best option. The cuts are closed using fine stitches, which may be dissolvable, and your breasts are wrapped in a special supportive dressing or support bra. You may also need to have drainage tubes fitted for up to 48 hours, to help drain away excess fluids.

**Breast implants improve the volume of the breasts and restore symmetry.**

## 3. THE RESULTS

The results of the procedure will be immediately obvious. While most women are pleased with how they look, they are not always as happy with how their breasts feel. You may have numbness in your nipple area, which is a common complication, or your breasts may feel supersensitive and painful to the touch. They may remain swollen and sensitive for a month or longer, though over time the swelling subsides and the incision lines will refine and fade.

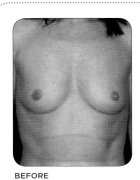

BEFORE

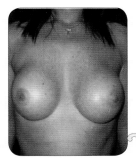

AFTER

# Recovery and healing

When you wake up you will feel tired, sore, and stiff, and will be advised to take painkillers. You may need a post-operative bra or compression bandage for extra support and positioning while you heal. Your breasts will be wrapped with gauze bandages as well as a tighter bandage for protection and support. Someone will need to drive you home, and you may need assistance over the next couple of days.

It takes a few months for the breasts to settle after surgery and, in the short term, you might experience some swelling, hardness, and discomfort along with some bruising, twinges, and pains over the first few weeks. The combination of increased volume from the breast implant and swelling from surgery may cause your breasts to feel large, heavy, and tight. You will be encouraged to rest in an upright position, to help reduce swelling.

Depending on the size of the breast implant and the way it was placed during surgery, some mild bruising may occur. Normal levels of bruising should subside in 1–2 weeks.

You will be given pain relief if needed. Your scars will be pink for several weeks, but will begin to fade after several months.

You will normally need to attend a number of post-operative check-ups to ensure that you are recovering well.

## Tips for a speedy recovery

- Rest—get as much as possible following your procedure. Drink plenty of fluids, and be sure to take your prescribed medications. Avoid sleeping on your front for 1 month.
- Avoid lifting your arms—for at least 3–5 days, you should try to keep arm extension to a minimum. The tissues will heal more quickly if you avoid stretching and separating muscle /tissue surrounding the implants.
- Take it easy—avoid physical exertion for several weeks and driving for 1 week. Breast implant recovery times vary from patient to patient and depend upon the technique, type of implant, and site of placement that the doctor uses, as well as the level of activities in your daily routine.
- Keep dry—avoid getting water on your wounds for a week.

# FACTS
## BREAST ENLARGEMENT

| | |
|---|---|
| **Description** | Surgery to increase the size of the breasts by inserting implants. |
| **Length of surgery** | 1–3 hours |
| **In/Outpatient** | Inpatient or outpatient |
| **Anesthesia** | General or intavenous sedation |
| **Back to work in...** | 2–4 weeks |
| **Back to the gym in...** | Several weeks |
| **Treatment frequency** | One or more times as desired |
| **Risks** | • For a few weeks after surgery, your breasts will feel sore, swollen, and hard, and you will feel a burning sensation in your nipples<br>• Scarring: pink and noticeable at first, but fading gradually<br>• An unevenness in size and shape—possibly caused by natural differences highlighted by the surgery<br>• Creasing, kinking, and ripples on the skin<br>• Infection<br>• Capsular contracture<br>• Change in skin and nipple sensation—may be permanent<br>• Seroma<br>• Unusual red or raised scars (keloids)—can take years to improve<br>• It's possible that you still won't be satisfied with your appearance after the operation |
| **Duration of results** | Long-lasting |

# BREAST REDUCTION
*Reduction mammoplasty*

## What is breast reduction?

**Large breasts can dominate a woman's appearance, give an unbalanced physical profile, and make exercise difficult or impossible. Overly large breasts often affect self-confidence, and even personal relationships. The aim of breast reduction surgery is to give smaller, shapelier breasts that are in proportion to the rest of the body.**

## WHY HAVE BREAST REDUCTION?

Breast reduction is a surgical procedure that brings the breasts into better proportion with the rest of the body by removing fat, excess breast tissue, and skin. The areola, or darker skin around the nipple, may be reduced and repositioned as well. Some breast reduction procedures are carried out in tandem with a breast lift; ideal for women who wish to improve the shape and the position of their breasts.

For many women (and men), it's not just the aesthetic issues they want to address; it is also about feeling physically better, as they experience problems such as back pain, neck pain, and skin irritations as well as even more serious issues like skeletal deformations and breathing problems. One problem is the bra straps, which make indentations in the skin. All of these factors can lead to feelings of self-consciousness.

Skin, fat, and glandular tissues are removed to make the breast smaller and lighter. You would be amazed at how little weight needs to come off to feel a big difference. Not only are the breasts smaller as a result,

but the darker skin around the nipples is reduced too in most cases.

Breast reduction for men, also known as gynecomastia, is a procedure for male patients who seek to correct overly large "breasts." (See page 198 for more information.)

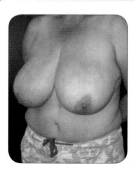
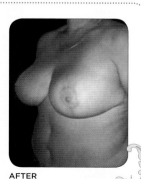

BEFORE

AFTER

# Am I a candidate for breast reduction surgery?

**Patients with any combination of these symptoms may be good candidates:**

- Women who have pendulous "sagging breasts" (this often signifies more glandular tissue than fat)
- Women who are thin (thin women tend to have more glandular tissue than fat)
- Women who have excessively large breasts (liposuction normally only provides a 30 to 50 percent reduction)
- Women who have excessively dense breast tissue (this often signifies more glandular tissue than fat)
- Women who have not yet reached the menopause (during the menopause fat replaces glandular tissue).

In most cases, breast reduction surgery cannot be performed until the breasts are fully grown, usually by age 18. A woman who intends to breastfeed a baby probably should not have the procedure. Women whose breasts are sagging but not too large might benefit more from a breast lift.

### WHAT TO EXPECT FROM A CONSULTATION WITH A BREAST REDUCTION SURGEON

During the consultation, your surgeon will take a detailed medical history, including whether or not you've ever had a lump removed from your breast or any other medical conditions affecting your breasts. He or she also will take a detailed family history. You should be in good physical and mental shape in order to undergo this surgery.

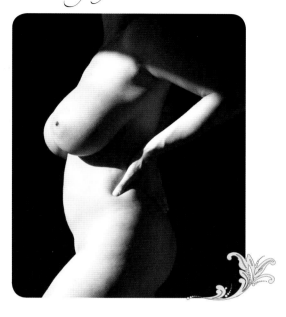

It is important that you are completely open as to why you're seeking a breast reduction. You should expect to discuss the emotional issues you've dealt with; that is, how have you felt, emotionally, about your breast size? How has it made you feel, physically? Has it caused any physical conditions?

Your surgeon may take photos of your breasts and measure them. During this time, he or she also will discuss how much breast tissue should be removed to achieve the desired results. You will also learn about how to prepare for the surgery and how to plan for your recovery. Your surgeon may prepare you for this procedure by performing a mammography and breast exam.

# The basic procedure

A breast reduction is usually performed through incisions made on your breasts with the surgical removal of the excess fat, glandular tissue, and skin. In some cases, excess fat may be removed by liposuction in conjunction with the excision techniques described below. Breast size is largely due to fatty tissue and excess skin is not a factor. Liposuction alone is not used for breast reduction. The technique used to reduce the size of your breasts will be determined by your individual condition, breast composition, the amount of reduction desired, your personal preferences, and your surgeon's professional advice.

## 1. ANESTHESIA

Medications are administered for your comfort during the surgical procedure. The choices include intravenous sedation and general anesthetic. Your surgeon will recommend the best one for you.

## 2. THE INCISIONS

**Incision options include:**

- A circular pattern around the areola: the incision lines that remain are visible and permanent scars, although usually well concealed beneath a swimsuit or bra
- A keyhole or racket-shaped pattern with an incision around the areola and vertically down to the breast crease
- An inverted T-/anchor-shaped incision.

## 3. REMOVAL OF TISSUE AND REPOSITIONING

After the incision is made, the nipple—which remains tethered to its original blood and nerve supply—is repositioned. The areola is reduced by excision of skin at the perimeter,

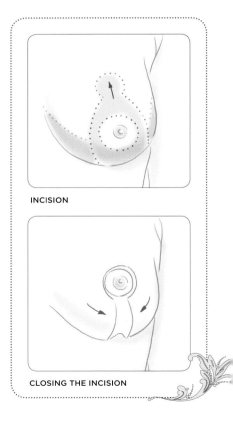

INCISION

CLOSING THE INCISION

if necessary. Underlying breast tissue is reduced, lifted, and shaped. Occasionally, for extremely large, pendulous breasts, the nipple and areola may need to be removed and transplanted to a higher position on the breast (free nipple graft).

## 4. CLOSING THE INCISIONS
The incisions are brought together to reshape the now smaller breast. Sutures are layered deep within the breast tissue to create and support the newly shaped breasts; sutures, skin adhesives, and/or surgical tape close the skin. Incision lines are permanent, but in most cases will fade and significantly improve over time.

## 5. THE RESULTS
The results of your breast reduction surgery will be immediately visible. Over time, post-surgical swelling will resolve and incision lines will fade. Satisfaction with your new image should continue to grow as you recover.

## Preparing for breast reduction surgery

Once you have made the decision to have breast reduction surgery, there are a number of steps that can help you prepare for the operation.

**Your surgeon will advise you to:**
- Avoid medications that may complicate surgery or recovery
- Stop smoking for a period of time before and after surgery
- Arrange for help or special care following surgery.

A breast reduction is usually performed under a general anesthetic. You will be asked not to eat or drink for about 6 hours beforehand; however, some anesthetists allow occasional sips of water until 2 hours before the operation.

You may also be asked to bring in a soft, supportive bra without underwiring to wear after surgery. Your surgeon will advise you about the most suitable type. Your nurse will explain how you will be cared for during your stay, and may do some tests. Your surgeon will usually visit you to discuss the operation and ask you to sign a consent form. He or she may draw on your breasts to show the planned size and shape. Photographs may also be taken, so that the results of surgery can be compared with your original appearance.

Your nurse will prepare you for theater. You may be asked to wear compression stockings to help prevent blood clots forming in the veins in your legs, and you will usually need to stay in hospital for 1–2 days post-op.

# Recovery and healing

After you are awakened and brought into the recovery room following your breast reduction surgery, the recovery nurse will monitor you until you are ready to be released. This is dependent upon the individual but may take up to 2 hours or more. You will feel quite tender and possibly confused as the anesthesia wears off.

A drain may be inserted to allow the fluids an exit from the incision sites or from the bottom portion of the treatment area. You will be swollen and bruised and will more than likely be wearing a type of compression garment or surgical bra with elastic bandages binding your breasts to your body.

It is important that you keep your incisions/suture line dry. Your surgeon may have placed adhesive strips on top of your incision line and sutures, or you may have internal sutures and tissue glue applied externally to bind your incision edges. Either way, your surgeon will give you specific care instructions. You will have your incision sites checked and your stitches removed in approximately 10 days.

While you are healing, take your temperature regularly. An elevated temperature could mean an infection. Pain tolerances depend upon the individual, but you will feel tender, stiff and sore for a few days and will more than likely not want to move too much. This will subside. Be sure to take your required medications and follow the precise instructions provided to you by your surgeon. As with all surgeries, swelling will be an issue. Swelling is a normal reaction to an injury and is categorized as a natural inflammatory action.

You may be swollen for 3 or 4 months, although this could be very slight and only noticed by you. Your breasts, of course, will be smaller than they were before, and higher, so you may not notice swelling, perhaps just soreness. Bruises may or may not be present.

Sleeping can be difficult initially; it is important to sleep with two or three fluffy pillows under your upper back and head to keep your torso elevated. This helps to relieve pressure on your treatment area, reducing swelling and pain. You should prepare for a period of several months to make a complete recovery from your breast reduction surgery.

## FACTS
**BREAST REDUCTION SURGERY**

| | |
|---|---|
| **Description** | Reduction of the breasts by removal of fat, tissue, and skin. |
| **Length of surgery** | 2–3 hours |
| **In/outpatient** | Inpatient |
| **Anesthesia** | General |
| **Back to work in...** | 1–2 weeks |
| **Back to the gym in...** | 1–2 months |
| **Treatment frequency** | Once |
| **Risks** | • Permanent scarring<br>• Post-surgical pain<br>• Breast asymmetry—after a breast reduction procedure, one breast may remain slightly larger than the other<br>• All breast reduction procedures carry a considerable risk that the woman will lose the ability to breastfeed. This is because most of the milk ducts in the breast are removed or otherwise altered during the surgical procedure. If your ability to breastfeed is important to you, a breast reduction may not be the right choice<br>• In rare cases, some (if not all) of the feeling in your breasts and/or nipples, can be lost, even after you are fully healed. While skilled, experienced surgeons are usually able to avoid damaging the blood vessels that nourish the breast nerve endings, there are no guarantees |
| **Duration of results** | Permanent |

# BREAST LIFT
## *Mastopexy*

## *What is a breast lift?*

A breast lift is a procedure to restructure breasts that have lost their original shape. Excess skin is removed and the surrounding tissue tightened to reshape and support the new breast contour. The areola can become enlarged over time and this can be corrected by a breast lift, too. The figure is rejuvenated with a profile that is more youthful, uplifted, and firm. Breast implants may also be inserted. A breast lift can also be appropriate for younger women who wish to address asymmetrical breasts.

### WHY HAVE A BREAST LIFT?

Over time a woman's breasts often change; many factors can bring about a loss of youthful shape and firmness, and of skin elasticity. These causes include: pregnancy, breastfeeding, weight fluctuations and weight gain, aging, and natural gravity—genes also have a lot to answer for. Breasts that have lost their once-firm uplifted contours can have a negative effect on a woman's self-confidence and self-image.

## *Am I a candidate for breast lift surgery?*

**You may be a candidate if you are:**

- At least 18 years of age
- A healthy individual not suffering from a life-threatening illness or any other medical condition that could impair healing and recovery
- A non-smoker
- Realistic in your expectations
- Not pregnant or breastfeeding.

It is also recomended that you should not be contemplating losing large amounts of weight after the surgery, as this can alter the appearance of the final results.

### WHAT TO EXPECT FROM A CONSULTATION WITH A BREAST LIFT SURGEON

You should have clear in your mind what you want to get out of your surgery. Your surgeon should go over in detail with you what the procedure can accomplish in your case, so you fully understand the realistic likely outcome of breast lift surgery.

# The basic procedure

A breast lift without implants is a highly individualized procedure achieved through a variety of incision patterns and techniques. The appropriate technique for your individual case will be determined by your breast size and shape, the size and the position of your areola, the degree of sagging, and your skin quality and elasticity, as well as the amount of extra skin.

## 1. ANESTHESIA

Medications are administered for your comfort during the procedure; the choices include intravenous sedation and general anesthesia. Your surgeon will recommend the best choice for you.

## 2. THE INCISIONS

The incision may include a circle around the areola, a line extending down the lower portion of the breast from the areola to the crease underneath the breast, or a line along the crease of the breast. Not every patient will require all of the incisions mentioned. It is possible to perform a breast lift through an incision around the areola only, or through a combination of incisions around the areola and a vertical incision down the lower portion of the breast.

## 3. RESHAPING AND SUTURING

Once the excess skin is removed, the breast tissue is reshaped and lifted and the remaining skin is tightened as the incisions are closed. Some incisions will be concealed in the natural breast contours; others are visible on the breast surface. Non-removable sutures are layered deep within the breast tissue to create and support the newly shaped breasts. Sutures, skin adhesives, and/or surgical tape may be used to close up the skin. Incision lines are permanent but in most cases fade and improve significantly with time.

## 4. THE RESULTS

The results are immediately visible. Over time, post-surgical swelling will subside and resolve, and incision lines will gradually refine in appearance. Patients often experience an immediate satisfaction with their results, with improved self-confidence and body image.

**Incisions may be made around the areola or vertically down the lower portion of the breast.**

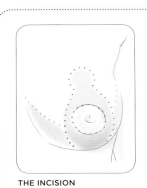

THE INCISION

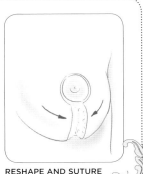

RESHAPE AND SUTURE

## Preparing for breast lift surgery

**Prior to surgery you may be asked to:**

- Get a lab testing or medical evaluation
- Take certain medications or adjust your current medications
- Get a baseline mammogram before surgery and perhaps after, too, to help detect any future changes in your breast tissue
- Stop smoking well in advance of surgery
- Avoid taking anti-inflammatory drugs, aspirin and herbal supplements as they may increase bleeding.

## Recovery and healing

After the procedure, the surgical areas will be covered in dressings or bandages and an elastic bandage or support bra will be given to you to wear to minimize swelling and support the breasts as they heal; you may have to wear the bra for the first week or two post-op.

Recovery times vary. There may be swelling and slight discomfort at the incision sites and in the breast tissue overall. It is quite common to experience discomfort, and this can be controlled with medication. A return to light and normal activity is possible a few days after surgery; sutures will be removed after 5–10 days. You will be able to return to work and resume normal activity after this time. It is advisable not to engage in any vigorous activity or heavy lifting for 4–6 weeks after your procedure.

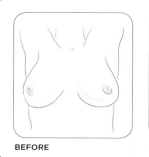

**BEFORE**

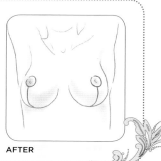

**AFTER**

## FACTS
### BREAST LIFT SURGERY

| | |
|---|---|
| **Description** | Restructuring of breasts that have lost their original shape. |
| **Length of surgery** | 1–3 hours |
| **In/outpatient** | Inpatient |
| **Anesthesia** | General or intravenous sedative |
| **Back to work in...** | 5–10 days |
| **Back to the gym in...** | 4–6 weeks |
| **Treatment frequency** | One or more times as desired |
| **Risks** | • Soreness, swelling, and burning sensation<br>• Scars: pink and noticeable at first, but fading gradually<br>• Dissatisfaction with results<br>• Hematoma<br>• Infection<br>• Poor healing of incisions<br>• Changes in nipples or breast sensation<br>• Skin discoloration, pigmentation changes, swelling, and bruising<br>• Damage to deeper structures such as nerves, blood vessels, muscles, and lungs<br>• Breast asymmetry<br>• Fluid accumulation<br>• Partial or total loss of feeling in the nipple or areola<br>• Blood clots<br>• Deep vein thrombosis, cardiac and pulmonary complications<br>• Pain |
| **Duration of results** | Long-lasting |

# BREAST RECONSTRUCTION

## WHY HAVE RECONSTRUCTION?

The aim of breast reconstruction is to create a soft, natural-looking breast for a woman who must undergo breast removal (mastectomy) or partial breast removal (lumpectomy) due to cancer or another disease, matching the remaining breast as closely as possible.

## What is breast reconstruction?

**There are two main ways of making a new breast. It can either be done by creating a breast "form" using an implant, which is put underneath the skin and muscle that covers the chest; or by using skin, fat, and sometimes muscle taken from another part of your own body.**

**Your surgeon will advise you on the type of breast reconstruction that is most suitable for you. It will depend on:**

- The amount of breast tissue that has been removed
- The healthiness of the tissue at the planned operation site
- Whether or not you have had radiotherapy to the breast area or chest wall
- Your general health and body build
- Your wishes and lifestyle.

The surgeon aims to create a breast similar in size and shape to your own breast. It is important to note that a reconstructed breast won't be identical to the existing breast, especially when naked. After your reconstruction, you may also need to have further surgery to create a nipple or to change the shape of your other breast to match the reconstructed one. It is possible to create a new nipple and this is usually done as a separate operation once the reconstructed breast has settled into its final shape. However, this is optional.

You can have reconstruction at the same time as your breast cancer surgery (immediate reconstruction) or later (delayed reconstruction). This is a personal decision—there is no right or wrong way.

# Am I a candidate for breast reconstruction surgery?

Almost every woman who has lost a breast to cancer or another illness can have her body restored with breast reconstruction surgery. However, the following conditions are desirable:

- As a candidate for breast reconstruction surgery it is important that you understand that although your figure will be significantly improved, your reconstructed breast will not look or feel exactly the same as the breast or breasts that were removed.
- Your oncologist has advised you that breast reconstruction is appropriate for you with regard to your cancer or treatment, and you have his or her full approval. (Should the cancer recur your reconstructed breast will not interfere with further treatment, however such treatment may affect the appearance of your reconstructed breast).

- You should feel ready to handle the period of emotional adjustment that may accompany breast reconstruction surgery. It will take time to adjust to a new reconstructed breast and accept it as your own.
- It is also important, when deciding to have breast reconstruction surgery, that you have no other additional health concerns that could complicate the procedure such as obesity or heart disease.

## WHAT TO EXPECT FROM A CONSULTATION WITH A BREAST RECONSTRUCTION SURGEON

To help determine which reconstruction method is best for you, your surgeon will perform a physical exam, during which he or she will take measurements and photographs for your medical record.

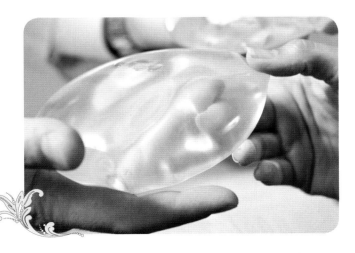

**Procedures using tissue expansion (see page 121) allow for the insertion of implants.**

# The basic procedure

Breast reconstruction usually involves more than one operation. The first stage, whether performed at the same time as the mastectomy or lumpectomy or later on, is typically performed in a hospital. Follow-up procedures may be performed in a hospital, an outpatient surgery center, or a surgical suite.

## 1. ANESTHESIA

Medications are administered for your comfort during the surgical procedure. The choices include intravenous sedation and general anesthetic. Your surgeon will recommend the best choice for you.

## 2. FLAP TECHNIQUES

Flap techniques reposition a woman's own muscle, fat, and skin to create or cover the breast mound. Sometimes a mastectomy or radiation therapy will leave insufficient tissue on the chest wall to cover and support a breast implant. The use of a breast implant for reconstruction almost always requires either a flap technique or tissue expansion.

- A TRAM flap uses donor muscle, fat, and skin from a woman's abdomen to reconstruct the breast. The flap may remain attached to the original blood supply and be tunneled up through the chest wall, or be completely detached, and formed into a breast mound.
- Alternatively, your surgeon may choose the DIEP or SGAP flap techniques, which do not use muscle but instead

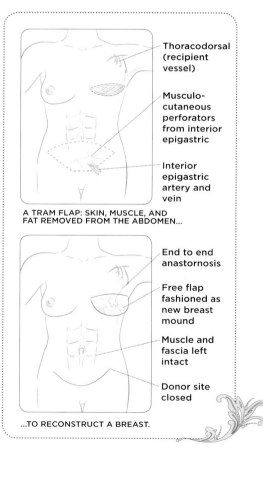

**Thoracodorsal (recipient vessel)**

**Musculo-cutaneous perforators from interior epigastric**

**Interior epigastric artery and vein**

A TRAM FLAP: SKIN, MUSCLE, AND FAT REMOVED FROM THE ABDOMEN...

**End to end anastornosis**

**Free flap fashioned as new breast mound**

**Muscle and fascia left intact**

**Donor site closed**

...TO RECONSTRUCT A BREAST.

transport tissue to the chest from the abdomen or buttock.

- A latissimus dorsi flap uses muscle, fat, and skin from the back tunneled to the mastectomy site, and remains attached to its donor site, leaving the blood supply intact.

Occasionally, the flap can reconstruct a complete breast mound, but more often it provides the muscle and tissue necessary to cover and support a breast implant.

### 3. TISSUE EXPANSION

Tissue expansion stretches healthy skin to provide coverage for a breast implant. Reconstruction with tissue expansion allows for an easier recovery than flap procedures, but it is a more lengthy reconstruction process. It requires many office visits, over 4–6 months after placement of the expander, to slowly fill the device through an internal valve and expand the skin. A second surgical procedure will be needed to replace the expander if it is not designed to serve as a permanent implant.

### 4. PLACING THE IMPLANT

A breast implant can be an addition or alternative to flap techniques. Saline and silicone implants are available for reconstruction. Your surgeon will help you decide what is best for you. Reconstruction with an implant alone usually requires tissue expansion.

### 5. GRAFTING

Grafting and other specialized techniques create a nipple (see right) and areola.

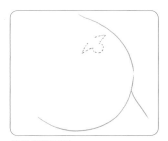

THE INCISION

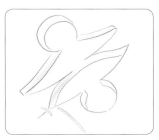

RAISING AND SUTURING

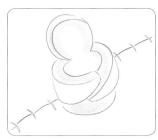

THE "NIPPLE" IS FORMED

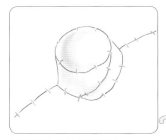

SUTURED INTO POSITION

# Recovery and healing

When the procedure is complete, you will be taken to a recovery area. Small drainage tubes may be placed beneath the skin near the surgical site to prevent fluids from accumulating. Recovering from a combined mastectomy and reconstruction or from a flap reconstruction typically takes longer than recovery from an implant reconstruction or a reconstruction performed apart from the mastectomy.

After the initial healing period you will return to your surgeon for a post-operative follow-up visit so that your healing and progress can be evaluated. You may find that sensation returns to some areas of the breast; however it is important to note that a reconstructed breast will never feel completely normal or have normal sensation. Breast reconstruction surgery can provide great physical and emotional rewards, and for many women it represents a chance to have a fresh start and put breast cancer and other illnesses behind them and get on with their lives. A period of some adjustment is quite normal for you to get used to your new look; any concerns about your new shape are likely to pass within a few months, as you begin to think of the reconstructed breast as your own.

**Breast reconstruction recovery times vary, but may follow this timeline:**

**Within 1 week:**
- Surgical drains (if used) will be removed and dressings will be changed
- Stitches will be removed.

**After 2 weeks:**
- Lingering soreness at the surgical sites usually tends to diminish
- You should start to feel less fatigued and regain some energy.

**After several weeks:**
- You should be able to return to most of your normal activities and routine, including sports and other physical activities
- You may begin stretching exercises under the guidance of your surgeon
- Your scars should start to fade, although it may take many months to see substantial fading.

# FACTS
## BREAST RECONSTRUCTION SURGERY

| | |
|---|---|
| **Description** | Creating a soft, natural-looking breast for a woman who must undergo breast removal. |
| **Length of surgery** | Varies: several hours |
| **In/outpatient** | Inpatient |
| **Anesthesia** | General |
| **Back to work in...** | 2 weeks |
| **Back to the gym in...** | 3–4 weeks |
| **Treatment frequency** | More than one operation required |
| **Risks** | • Bleeding<br>• Fluid collection with swelling and pain<br>• Excessive scar tissue<br>• Infection<br>• Tissue necrosis (death) of all or part of the flap<br>• Problems at the donor site (immediate and long-term)<br>• Changes in nipple and breast sensation<br>• Fatigue<br>• The need for additional surgeries to correct problems<br>• Changes in the nearby arm |
| **Duration of results** | Permanent |

# BREAST AUGMENTATION REVISION

## What is the procedure?

**The most common reasons for breast implant removal surgery include: implant leakage or rupture, capsular contracture, a change in size or shape, or dissatisfaction with the results of surgery. Some women experience complications after breast augmentation, such as asymmetry, breast pain, and deflation. Fortunately, it is possible to correct most complications with the removal or replacement of implants.**

### WHY HAVE BREAST REVISION?

Breast implant revision, also referred to as breast augmentation revision or breast revision, is a cosmetic surgery procedure involving the removal and/or replacement of breast implants to correct complications that have occurred after breast augmentation or implant-based breast reconstruction surgery. Breast implant revision can also be performed to correct an unsatisfactory result from either of the surgeries mentioned.

## How is a breast revision procedure performed?

For implant removal surgery, general anesthesia or intravenous sedation is normally used. An incision is made either around the areola or under the fold of the breast. The capsule around the implant is cut into and the implant is carefully removed. If the implant is silicone-filled, it is inspected for any signs of damage and rupture before removal. If the implant is filled with saline, the surgeon may choose to deflate the implant to help removal. The implants are then replaced with new ones. The scar tissue (capsule) that was around the implant may also be removed (if the implant is not going to be replaced).

If the surgical procedure consists only of removing the old implants, then pain will be minimal. If implants and capsules are removed, the discomfort will be similar to the discomfort experienced after a standard breast augmentation procedure.

You should be pain-free until the day after your surgery. If you experience some discomfort, prescription pain medication will be available to you. You may be asked to take antibiotics and other medications as necessary.

## SIDE EFFECTS AND RISKS

Like all surgical procedures, with breast implant removal surgery there is always a possibility of complications. Although these complications are extremely rare, they can include:

- Infection
- Adverse reaction to the anesthesia
- Excessive bleeding
- Unsatisfactory results

Breast asymmetry may occur after breast implant removal surgery if the implant is not replaced. It is important to bear in mind that you may be disappointed with the results of breast implant removal surgery. Additional surgery may be necessary to reshape breasts after implant removal.

Some patients require no further surgery after their implants have been removed, while others may require a breast lift. Breast lift surgery can leave scars on the outside of the breasts, which will heal in time.

If the implant shell has been damaged or ruptured, it may be impossible to remove all of the escaped gel from the surrounding tissues. This is a particular problem if the surrounding scar capsule, which usually contains the leaked gel, has also been injured or damaged.

It is not possible to predict with certainty how a woman will look after implant removal surgery. Much depends on the nature of the scar capsule and whether the implant has ruptured.

## Recovery and healing

Recovery and healing times vary. Your stitches would normally be removed 5–7 days post surgery. Bruising subsides gradually over 2–3 weeks. You should walk around the house with some assistance. Every day, walk around the house, slowly increasing your level of activity. Avoid raising your shoulders above 90 degrees for 2 weeks. If you have small children try to arrange for their care by your spouse or another guardian for the first few days. You will need to avoid reaching or lifting of any kind for at least a week and maybe as long as 2 weeks. Although it is important to keep the breast area clean throughout the healing process to avoid infections, breast implant removal patients should not submerge their incisions in a bath, swimming pool, or other body of water until the breasts have completely healed. Avoid touching the incisions or bringing any product, such as lotion or deodorant, into contact with the stitched area. You should be able to return to work after a week. However, if your job requires physical activity, you should wait 2 weeks before resuming a full workload. It may take your body up to 6 weeks to make a full recovery. As your body heals, you will gradually regain strength of movement. Your scars may take up to 7 months to completely heal.

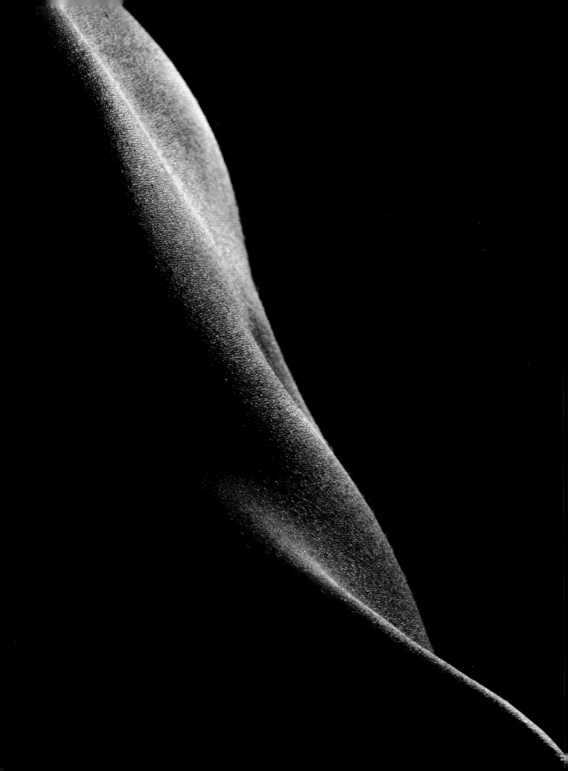

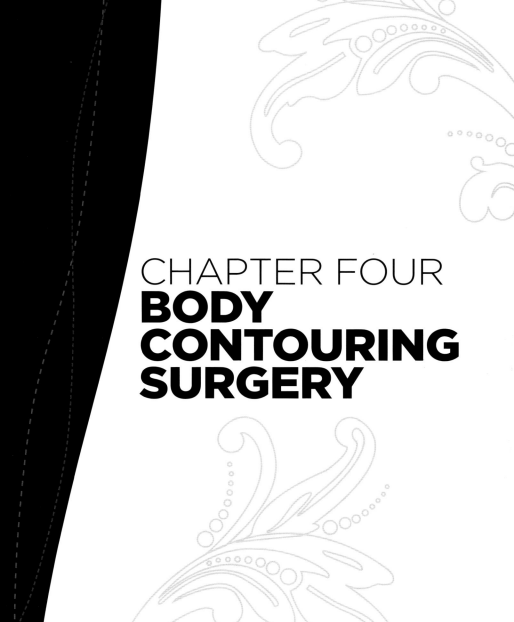

# CHAPTER FOUR
# BODY CONTOURING SURGERY

# BODY CONTOURING SURGERY
*An overview*

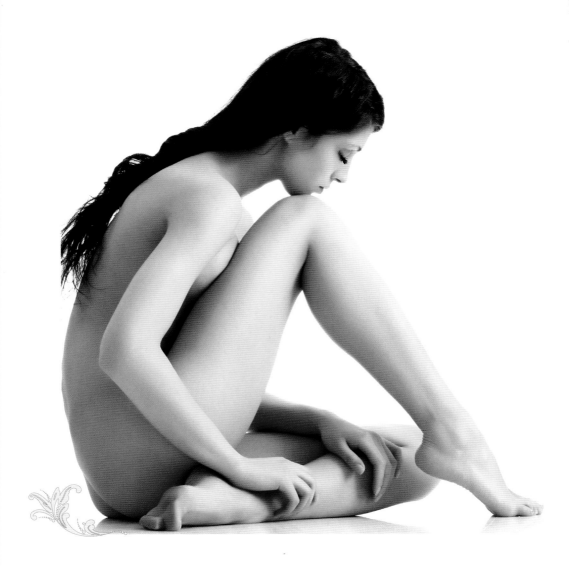

Cosmetic surgery for the body covers a number of surgical procedures that reduce or alter the shape and size of areas of the body including the arms, abdomen, buttocks, thighs, and calves. Procedures also include surgery to improve the function and appearance of parts of the body that have been damaged by injury, for example, the hands. Body-contouring surgery, as its name suggests, specifically includes all those operations designed to improve the overall shape and tone of the body.

Body-contouring procedures can include the following:
- Fat removal (liposculpture, liposuction, male chest reduction)
- Skin tightening (abdominoplasty; arm, thigh, and buttock lifts)
- Muscle enhancing (abdominal muscle plication; calf, buttock, and pectoral implants; abdominal six-pack etching).

## LIPOSUCTION
One of the most popular cosmetic surgery treatments sought by both women and men is liposuction. Liposuction is the surgical cosmetic procedure for reducing fat deposits that are resistant to diet and exercise; literally by removing fat.

## TUMMY TUCK (ABDOMINOPLASTY)
Tummy tuck surgery is a procedure used to give a tighter, flatter stomach. Frequent changes in weight, aging, and life in general can make the stomach muscles weaken, the skin sag, and stretch marks appear. Abdominoplasty flattens the slack skin and tightens the muscles of the relaxed tummy wall, and if needed, excess subcutaneous fatty tissue can be removed as well. Tummy tuck surgery not only results in a better appearance, but it also stops the slackening process of the abdominal wall. The abdominoplasty procedure is not a substitute for physical exercise and a balanced diet and cannot help weight control. However, the results can be long-lasting, especially if you exercise, eat a healthy diet, and maintain a healthy weight after your operation.

## BUTTOCK IMPLANTS (GLUTEAL AUGMENTATION)
The buttock implant procedure is the surgical insertion of artificial implants into the buttocks in order to enhance their size and shape. Buttock implants are used to make the buttocks larger and shapelier, and can also provide individuals with underdeveloped buttocks with a more proportionate figure.

## BUTTOCK LIFT (GLUTEOPLASTY)

The buttock lift (gluteoplasty) is a surgical procedure to remove excess fat and loose skin in the buttock area and may be combined with liposuction to further improve the body contours. The buttock lift procedure involves cutting the skin high up on the side of the thigh and buttocks, removing excess fat, and trimming away the excess skin. Liposuction and buttock implants may be used at the same time to create the desired result.

## THIGH LIFT AND REDUCTION

Thigh lift is a surgical procedure done to tighten sagging muscles and remove excess skin in the thigh area. Thigh lift surgery can be performed in conjunction with other procedures, such as a body lift. Thigh reduction surgery removes excess skin and fat from the inside and the outside of the upper thigh. The surgery leaves a long, noticeable scar. Thigh reduction improves the body contour in clothes, but the scars are visible in underwear or swimwear.

## UPPER ARM LIFT (BRACHIOPLASTY)

An upper arm lift is a surgical procedure that reshapes the underneath portion of the upper arm to reduce excess sagging skin, remove fat, and smooth and tighten the appearance of the upper arm. During the procedure, excess skin, underlying tissue, and fat are removed between the underarm and the elbow, and the remaining skin and tissue are lifted to achieve a tighter, smoother, and uplifted effect.

## CALF AUGMENTATION AND IMPLANTS

Calf augmentation creates cosmetic fullness in the lower leg. It corrects muscle imbalance as a result of both physical and congenital defects such as "skinny/chicken" legs, bowed legs, clubfoot, or disproportionate calf development. Calf implants, made of soft, solid silicone, are placed in "pockets" overlying the existing muscles. One or two calf implants may be inserted, depending on the desired effect. The existing muscles in the calf area are made to appear larger and more defined.

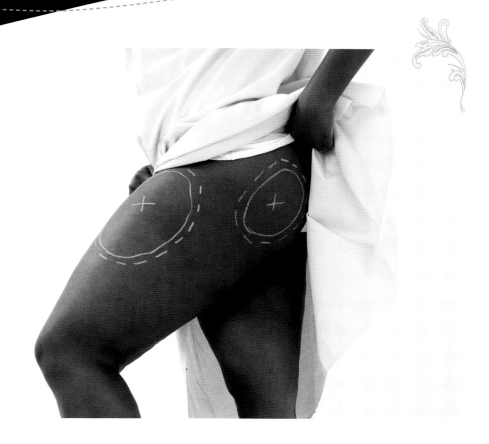

## HOW DO I DECIDE WHICH TREATMENTS TO HAVE?

- If there is localized fat: liposculpture is the answer.
- If there is excess skin: some form of lift or tuck is required.
- If there is poor muscle definition: exercise and/or muscle-enhancing surgery is needed.
- If the appearance of the skin is the issue: a number of options are available.

For any one anatomical area of the body, one or more procedures might be necessary (e.g. both fat removal and skin tightening on a fat saggy abdomen). Similarly, for any one patient, a combination of procedures might be recommended for different areas (e.g. skin tightening to the arms, liposculpture to the hips, and so on).

# LIPOSUCTION
## *Lipoplasty*

**Since the invention of liposuction in Italy in the early 1970s and its refinement and development by American doctors in the 1980s, the procedure of permanently removing fat deposits using a high-pressured vacuum device has been gaining in popularity.**

Liposuction is a surgical cosmetic procedure for reducing fat deposits that are resistant to diet and exercise; literally removing fat and re-sculpting the body. A cannula is used to break up and suck out this fat from the body.

The best candidates for liposuction surgery are at least 18 years of age, psychologically stable, and in good physical health. There is an increased risk of surgical complications if there is a medical history of immunodeficiency disorders, cardiac problems, seizure disorders, excessive bleeding, or a significant history of deep vein thrombosis. Also, certain drugs increase the risk of bleeding, such as anti-inflammatory drugs or anticoagulants, and if you were taking these then liposuction would not be a safe procedure.

When considering a liposuction, you will have an initial consultation with your surgeon to discuss the changes that you would like to make to your appearance. He or she will explain the options available to you, the risks and limitations, as well as the cost. It is important to ask questions to help you make an informed decision.

Liposuction surgery is always performed under anesthetic; usually general, but occasionally local or regional if only a small area is being treated. A conventional liposuction treatment or a variation of it such as tumescent liposuction will usually take 1–2 hours per area treated, but longer procedures such as large-volume liposuction can take much longer, and may even require several procedures.

Once the procedure is complete, swelling should subside within three weeks and, to aid the healing process, your surgeon will probably tell you to begin light activity as soon as possible. Liposuction recovery times vary, however you should be able to return to work after three days to three weeks, depending on the extent of surgery, and normal activities including exercise can be resumed in 4 to 6 weeks.

Although conventional liposuction is the most commonly performed cosmetic surgery procedure in the U.S., and the majority of operations are successful, there are risks, as with any surgery. Some patients experience side effects, and it is possible that follow-up surgery may be required.

Liposuction permanently removes a portion of the fat cells and so patients tend not to regain weight in that area, making it a very desirable surgical procedure.

# Types of liposuction

## CONVENTIONAL LIPOSUCTION

This is the classic liposuction treatment, and is the removal of fat from under the skin using a strong suction device that literally pulls the unwanted fat cells out of the body. This causes the skin to shrink to the newly contoured body accordingly, leaving a new, slimmer, re-sculpted body.

## TUMESCENT LIPOSUCTION

Tumescent liposuction involves large volumes of saline solution being injected into the fat deposits prior to surgery, making them easier to break up and then extract, for more enhanced results.

## LARGE-VOLUME LIPOSUCTION

Large-volume liposuction involves circumferential body contouring, with at least five body areas being treated in one single operation. According to the American Society of Plastic Surgery, any liposuction procedure in which more than 10 pints (5 liters) of fluid and fat is removed is classified as large-volume liposuction. The procedure can sculpt the body to a curvaceous form and help you to take off many inches of waist.

## ULTRASONIC LIPOSUCTION

Ultrasonic liposuction uses sound-wave vibrations to rupture fat cells and thus liquefy the fat, making it easier to dislodge during suction. This process leads to increased vascularization of cells, and a newer and thicker band of collagen is formed in the upper layers of skin, causing a smoother appearance and surface in areas of skin that were formerly textured with cellulite.

Ultrasonic liposuction can also be performed as non-invasive liposuction, also known as laser lipolysis or laser liposuction. This involves several sessions of over a period of a few months to achieve a smoother contour without having invasive surgery.

Laser Lypo is a procedure that uses an ultrafine and flexible cannula; no vacuum suction is performed, so the trauma to the body is light. The incision made in the skin is so tiny that stitching is not required. After a local anesthetic injection, the laser is inserted into the layer of fat just underneath the skin and moved around in slow, fanning movements. The heat it produces destroys the walls of the fat cells and liquefies the fat within them, while sealing off blood vessels, which minimizes internal bleeding and bruising. Depending on the number of areas treated, the procedure can take from 20 minutes to 2½ hours.

# CONVENTIONAL LIPOSUCTION

## What is conventional liposuction?

The liposuction process involves the insertion of a cannula through a small incision concealed in a skin fold near the site to be reduced; the scars are virtually undetectable. Through repeated movements of the cannula under the skin, fat globules are separated and removed by vacuum suction through the cannula. Usually only one small incision will be needed for each area being treated with conventional liposuction. The area concerned is injected with various solutions prior to insertion of the cannula to reduce bleeding and to assist the breakdown of the fat globules.

### WHY HAVE CONVENTIONAL LIPO?

Conventional liposuction helps both men and women to improve the contours of their bodies, through a relatively simple and safe surgical procedure.

Liposuction sculpts or re-contours the body, but does not necessarily result in weight loss. The aim of conventional liposuction surgery is to lose inches rather than weight, and to alter the patient's shape. It is very effective in the removal of unwanted bumps and bulges and in improving the body's silhouette.

### Areas of the body that benefit from conventional liposuction:

- Cheeks, jowls, and neck
- Upper arms
- Breast or chest areas
- Back
- Abdomen and waistline
- Hips and buttocks
- Inner and outer thighs
- Knees, calves, and ankles.

Conventional liposuction surgery can be combined with other cosmetic surgery techniques and may be carried out in a number of areas at the same time. The amount of fat removed varies, but between 2–4 pints (1–2 liters) is considered safe. Fat cells removed by conventional liposuction are permanently removed and fat cannot be laid down again in the area that has been treated. However, you will still gain weight if you overeat, though the fat will show in other areas.

# Am I a candidate for conventional liposuction?

If you are considering liposuction, it is important that you have realistic expectations. Although dramatic results can be achieved, they may not be as immediate or obvious as you would like. The success of liposuction surgery, as with all cosmetic procedures, depends on a number of individual factors, such as age, skin elasticity, weight, and overall health.

The ideal liposuction candidate is someone within 30–40 lb (15–20 kg) of their ideal body weight with localized problem areas of fat. Your BMI (body mass index), which is a measurement of your total fat content in relation to your size, will be assessed. This gives a baseline for the liposuction surgeon to use to determine your suitability for the procedure.

**Before undergoing conventional liposuction, ask yourself:**
- Have I tried diet and exercise?
- Am I of normal weight for my height?
- Am I in generally good health?
- Is my excess fat in specific areas?
- Does my skin have reasonably good elasticity?

**Liposuction is not suitable for people with:**
- A weakened immune system
- Diabetes
- Heart or artery problems
- A history of blood clots or restricted blood flow.

Liposuction surgery cannot be used to treat obesity, and will also not necessarily eliminate cellulite.

## WHAT TO EXPECT FROM A CONSULTATION WITH A LIPOSUCTION SURGEON

During the consultation, your surgeon will be able to educate you on the possible risks and complications involved in liposuction surgery. The surgeon will be able to suggest the liposuction procedure that will address your specific body issues.

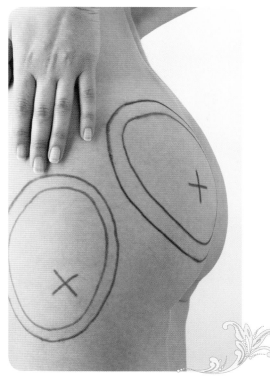

# The basic procedure

## 1. ANESTHESIA

The liposuction procedure is performed under a general or twilight (where you are sedated but not unconscious) anesthetic, depending on the type and number of liposuction procedures you undergo. The liposuction operation is often performed as a day case, taking approximately 1–2 hours, though you may need to stay in the hospital overnight.

The surgical liposuction process often involves the injection of a numbing solution. With a local anesthesia, your doctor will only numb the area of your body being treated, and you will be conscious during the liposuction surgery. General anesthesia can be administered either as a gas or through a needle injection, and will put you to sleep for the operation. Once you awaken, you will still be numb in the area of the body that has been treated, and will feel little or no pain.

## 2. THE INCISIONS

After administering the anesthesia and, if needed, injecting fluids, the next step is to create tiny incisions in the area of the body from which fat deposits will be removed. These incisions are usually quite small, 1/3 in (1 cm) long at most. These incisions are then used to insert the cannula, a thin vacuum tube, which will extract the fat.

## 3. FAT REMOVAL

The surgeon will insert the cannula through the incision (or incisions), into the deep fat layer beneath your skin. Using backward and forward movements, the surgeon uses the cannula to break up and suction away the unwanted fat deposits beneath the skin. A significant amount of blood and other bodily fluids are removed along with

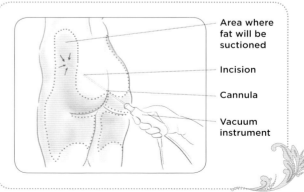

Area where fat will be suctioned

Incision

Cannula

Vacuum instrument

**Small incisions are made which are then used to insert a cannula to extract the fat.**

**The surgeon inserts the cannula into the deep fat layer of the skin to break up and suction away unwanted fat.**

the fat, so you will be given replacement fluids intravenously during and after the liposuction procedure and in recovery.

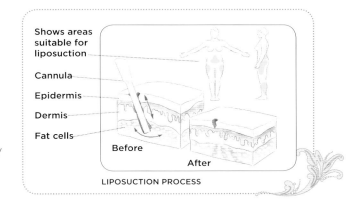

Shows areas suitable for liposuction

Cannula

Epidermis

Dermis

Fat cells

Before

After

LIPOSUCTION PROCESS

## 4. CLOSING THE INCISIONS

When the fat-removal part of the liposuction procedure is complete, the incisions can either be closed with a few stitches or left open. This normally depends on your surgeon's preference, though leaving the incisions open can reduce the amount of bruising and swelling that take place after a liposuction operation.

## *Preparing for conventional liposuction surgery*

If you are on the birth control pill, stop taking it and use another birth control method until after the surgery. This is necessary to reduce the risk of blood clots in your legs after surgery. Avoid aspirin, ibuprofen, and other non-steroidal anti-inflammatory drugs for 7 to 10 days before surgery. These drugs may contribute to bleeding during and after surgery. Some vitamins and herbs also affect bleeding, so ask your doctor which nutritional supplements to avoid. If you smoke, stop smoking before surgery and don't resume afterward. Smokers risk chest infections after anesthesia. Smoking also reduces the blood flow to the skin, which can increase the risk of circulation problems after surgery.

If you lose weight before your liposuction, lose only as much weight as you can honestly keep off later. A large weight gain soon after surgery could negatively affect your results.

Liposuction usually takes place on an outpatient basis, allowing you to go home the same day of surgery. However, you may need to plan for a hospital stay if a large amount of fat is to be removed or other procedures are to be done at the same time. Make sure you have someone who can drive you home after the surgery and stay with you for the first day.

# Recovery and healing

The results of the procedure will be immediately noticeable. There is often some bruising and swelling; however this should subside after 1–2 weeks. It is advisable to take 1–2 weeks off work, depending on the nature of your job. The areas affected by the surgery will be swollen, sore, and tender to the touch for up to 3 months after surgery. You will be required to wear a support garment for up to 6 weeks after your liposuction operation. The appearance of the treated areas will continue to improve once swelling subsides, and your unwanted fat will be gone, resulting in a slimmer, smoother body contour.

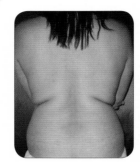 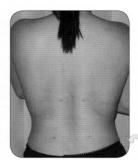

BEFORE                    AFTER

Liposuction recovery times vary from procedure to procedure. For instance, if you are having lipoplasty surgery on your face, the recovery time will be a lot longer than it would be if you were having surgery on your limbs. Recovery times are also dependent on how much fat has been removed, and how large the area is.

After liposuction surgery, there is always some fluid left beneath the skin. If the incisions are stitched shut, the fluid drains less easily and this can lead to bruising or swelling. You will need to wear compression bandages or a compression suit for about 1 month after your liposuction surgery. Compression bandages and suits are necessary to compress the areas that have been treated, encourage proper draining of fluid, and make it easier for your body to heal into its new shape. Fluid buildup is a common after-effect of liposuction surgery. Drains, inserted just beneath the skin, may sometimes be temporarily used to drain any excess blood or fluid. These can be uncomfortable, but are essential to ensure that you heal properly after your liposuction procedure. Your doctor may prescribe antibiotics to prevent infection.

You can expect to really see your new body shape about 3 months after your liposuction surgery, and it is important that you continue to eat healthily and exercise to maintain your new figure.

# FACTS
## CONVENTIONAL LIPOSUCTION

| | |
|---|---|
| **Description** | Fat is removed from specific areas of the body. |
| **Length of surgery** | Varies: from 1–2 hours per area treated |
| **In/outpatient** | Inpatient or outpatient |
| **Anesthesia** | General or twilight |
| **Back to work in...** | Varies |
| **Back to the gym in...** | Varies |
| **Treatment frequency** | One or more times as desired |
| **Risks** | • Bruising<br>• Swelling<br>• Discomfort<br>• Infection<br>• Numbness—may be temporary or permanent<br>• Extended healing time<br>• Blood clots—can migrate to the lungs and lead to death<br>• Irregularities in the skin—it may appear bumpy or withered due to uneven fat removal, poor skin elasticity, and incorrect healing<br>• An allergic reaction to the medication or anesthesia<br>• Scarring<br>• Excessive fluid loss—can lead to shock and, in some cases, death<br>• Accumulation of fluid<br>• Nerve damage<br>• Damage to vital organs |
| **Duration of results** | Long-lasting |

# TUMESCENT LIPOSUCTION
## Tumescent liposculpting

## What is a tumescent liposuction?

**The tumescent liposuction advantage is two-fold: first; it only requires local anesthesia, and second it is minimally invasive, requiring only a few tiny incisions. Those factors reduce the recovery time to approximately 24–48 hours. All surgical liposuction techniques are meant to improve the body's contour by removing fat deposits located between the skin and muscle, but the tumescent liposuction technique can do this much more accurately and remove more of the fat layer. With this surgical procedure the** patient is usually awake, which allows the surgeon to feel the patient's muscle tone alongside the fat layer. This is a huge advantage as it lets a surgeon experienced in the tumescent technique extract more fat than by tradition liposuction methods.

### WHY HAVE TUMESCENT LIPO?

Tumescent liposuction is a popular and effective method of liposuction. Although it is relatively new in the world of cosmetic surgery, it has become extremely popular because of its combination of safety and accuracy.

## Body areas that can be treated:

- Neck and jowls
- Arms
- Abdomen
- Buttocks
- Hips
- Inner and outer thighs ("saddlebags" on women)
- Knees
- Legs
- Flanks ("love handles" on men)
- Enlarged male breasts (gynecomastia). Tumescent liposuction can be combined with other liposuction techniques. Often other liposuction modalities are performed first to loosen the fat and then the surgeon removes what is left through the tumescent liposuction technique.

# Am I a candidate for tumescent liposuction surgery?

A good candidate for liposuction is one who has realistic expectations for the outcome, is in good physical and mental health. Liposuction is not for those on certain medical treatments and medications.

**The best candidates for liposuction meet the following criteria:**

- They are in good mental and physical health
- They are within 25 lb (12 kg) of their ideal weight
- They have firm, elastic skin
- They are not prone to weight fluctuations
- They have no significant medical problems such as diabetes, heart or lung disease, or poor circulation
- They do not smoke
- They are well informed about the liposuction procedure
- They have realistic expectations
- They exercise regularly.

You should also bear in mind that liposuction should not be considered a weight-loss technique or a solution to obesity.

## WHAT TO EXPECT FROM A CONSULTATION WITH A TUMESCENT LIPOSUCTION SURGEON

During your consultation you will be asked a number of questions about your health, and lifestyle. Your surgeon may:

- Evaluate your general health status and any pre-existing health conditions or risk factors
- Examine and measure your body, including taking detailed measurements
- Take photographs for your medical records and post-op assessment
- Discuss the options and recommend the best procedure for your objectives and goals
- Discuss likely outcomes of liposuction surgery and any risks or potential complications.

**Tumescent liposuction improves the contour of the body.**

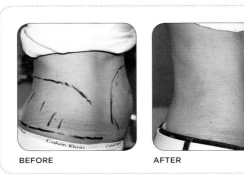

BEFORE          AFTER

# How is tumescent liposuction performed?

Tumescent liposuction patients do not need general anesthesia. Most patients receive no sedation or only minor sedation to help them relax and are completely comfortable and awake during the tumescent liposuction surgery.

Cannulas have now been miniaturized so that they can be inserted through much smaller openings in the skin. A number of small holes may be made in the skin around the area to be treated (instead of fewer, larger holes). The cannula is attached to a powerful vacuum, which removes the fat. As the procedure continues, the cannula is moved to other areas where it tunnels into the fat until the necessary amount is removed.

Your surgeon will mark the treatment area on your body. Photographs may be taken, so that the results of liposuction can be compared with your original appearance.

# Recovery and healing

Recovery usually takes 3 weeks. Most patients feel some bruising and swelling in the treated areas. Post-operative pain is well controlled by anesthetics used in tumescent surgery as well as prescribed painkillers. Patients may resume work, light exercise, and physical activity within the first 2 days after the procedure. They may get back to their normal physical routine within the first few weeks. Patients may return to work within 2 days after surgery.

If a patient remains active and follows a reasonable diet, the surgery results are there to stay for a very long time.

## SIDE EFFECTS AND RISKS

Although tumescent liposuction is a safe procedure, just as with any surgery it may carries certain risks and possible complications. These risks are the same as for patients undergoing standard liposuction (see pages 138 to 139). If greater areas are treated or bigger amounts of fatty fluid are extracted, then the risk of complications increases. Most of these risks are diminished if a specialized and qualified board-certified surgeon performs this surgical procedure; however, even then complications may occur.

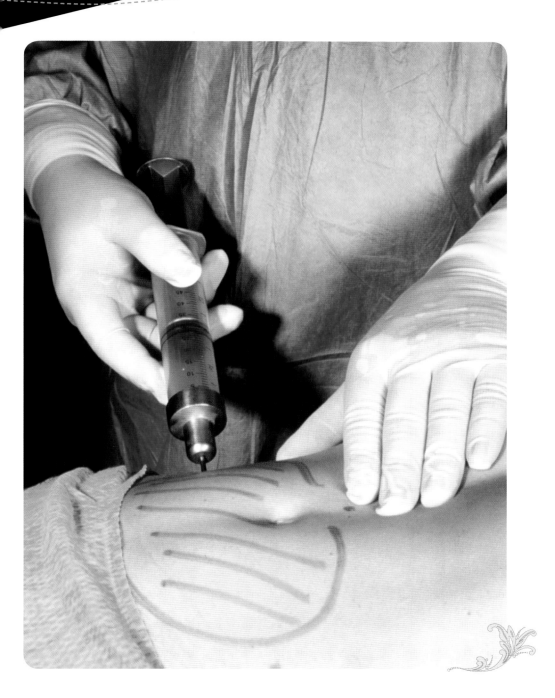

# ULTRASONIC LIPOSUCTION
## Ultrasound-assisted lipoplasty

Ultrasonic liposuction can be done on your abdomen, hips, thighs, the insides of the knees, ankles, upper arms, neck, and back. It can also be performed on areas that have been previously treated with liposuction but are in need of further contouring. It is not a treatment for weight-control or obesity, and it can't remove cellulite or stretch marks.

## What is ultrasonic liposuction?

**Ultrasonic liposuction is a form of liposuction that uses ultrasonic soundwaves to "melt" fat deposits into a liquid state. This liquefied fat is combined with a special fluid that causes it to emulsify, making its removal much easier.**

**Ultrasound liposuction surgery has advantages over traditional surgery. These advantages include:**

- Less trauma to adjacent organs
- Smaller incisions
- More precise control in surgery
- Minimal tissue handling
- Reduced blood loss
- Reduced risk of infection
- Less post-op pain
- Less scarring
- Reduced risk of wound complications.

There are other benefits associated with ultrasonic liposuction fat removal, including the ability to treat areas that have denser fat deposits and to remove larger volumes of fat at one time. Ultrasonic liposuction also tightens the skin during the process. It is often used after regular (tumescent) liposuction to achieve a finer, more precise result.

However, this type of liposuction is also associated with an increased risk of complications compared to conventional liposuction, such as burning and/or tingling, swelling, skin burns, and seromas (where fluid collects under the skin).

# Am I a candidate for ultrasonic liposuction?

The procedure is most suited to those who are close to their ideal body weight, but if you have a lot of fat in an isolated area, you may still be a good candidate. Some patients find liposuction to be a good incentive for weight loss, but it is not a treatment for weight control or obesity.

**You may be a good candidate if:**

- You would like to remove specific areas of fat that are diet- and exercise-resistant
- You have realistic expectations
- You have good skin tone and elasticity
- You have no loose or saggy skin
- You are within 30 percent of your ideal body weight
- Your weight has been stable for six months or more
- You are emotionally stable.

Good skin tone is a prerequisite for ultrasonic liposuction. Saggy skin or stretch marks will affect the quality of the results, and may look worse.

### WHAT TO EXPECT FROM A CONSULTATION WITH AN ULTRASONIC LIPOSUCTION SURGEON

You will be asked to describe in detail what you would like improve. Your surgeon needs to fully understand your needs to determine whether your desired outcome is realistic. Your overall weight, skin and muscle tone, and the distribution of fat deposits will determine which techniques will be used and what results can be achieved.

Weight loss is often recommended prior to surgery to enhance the result. If multiple areas are to be treated, your surgeon may recommend more than one operation, a month or two apart.

# The basic procedure

## 1. ANESTHESIA

Liposuction can be performed under general anesthetic, where you are completely asleep, or under sedation, where you are not unconscious but are very relaxed and in a light sleep. Your doctor will discuss your options, depending on how many areas are being worked on.

## 2. INCISIONS AND LIPOSUCTION

Small incisions are made in the areas to be treated. The cannula contains an ultrasonic probe at the end and is attached to an ultrasonic generator and a suction vacuum. Tumescent fluid (a mixture of anesthetic, saline solution, and epinephrine) is added through the incisions into the fat to be removed—this fluid swells the skin and allows the surgeon easier access to the area. The cannula is then inserted through the incision and passed through the fat. The soundwave energy generated by the cannula breaks up the fat cells and converts them to oil (emulsifies them). The oil mixes with the fluid and is easily vacuumed out.

### 3. CLOSING THE INCISIONS

When all the fat has been vacuumed out, the incisions are closed. The treated areas will be strapped with bandages, and a snug elastic dressing, support girdle, or body stocking must be worn over the treated area to control swelling and bleeding, aid healing, and help your skin shrink to fit your new shape. You may need to wear this garment continuously for 2–3 weeks, then just in the daytime for a few more weeks, depending on your surgeon's instructions. You may also have a small drainage tube inserted under the skin to prevent fluid from accumulating.

### 4. THE RESULTS

The length of time until the post-operative swelling has decreased and the permanent results become visible depends on the surgeon's technique and how many areas were worked on. The new shape of your body should begin to emerge in the first few weeks, though swelling may still be present for several months. The final result of your surgery should be clearly seen after about 6 months.

## Recovery and healing

The areas that were treated will be bruised and tender for several weeks. Some swelling will remain for several months, and your size may actually get larger before it gets smaller. Most people return to normal after 2 weeks and experience optimal results over the next several months.

During the first few weeks most people experience varying degrees of pain, burning, swelling, and temporary numbness. You will be advised to wear compression garments for several days.

After a few weeks, you should feel comfortable enough to remove the compression garment. The skin surrounding the treated area may seem loose, but it will tighten within about 6 months. Your surgeon may schedule check-ups to monitor your healing; recovery time will vary depending on the amount of fat removed.

# FACTS
## ULTRASONIC LIPOSUCTION

| | |
|---|---|
| **Description** | Ultrasonic liposuction is a form of liposuction that uses ultrasonic soundwaves to "melt" fat deposits. |
| **Length of surgery** | Varies: from 1–2 hours per area treated |
| **In/outpatient** | Inpatient or outpatient |
| **Anesthesia** | General or twilight |
| **Back to work in...** | 1–2 weeks |
| **Back to the gym in...** | 3–4 weeks |
| **Treatment frequency** | Once |
| **Risks** | • Bruising, swelling, and scarring<br>• Thrombophlebitis—inflammation of the veins may occur but should settle after a few weeks<br>• Swollen ankles<br>• Seroma<br>• Hematoma<br>• Pulmonary embolism—can be fatal<br>• Numbness—temporary or permanent<br>• Damage to internal organs<br>• Disruption of the fluid balance of the body<br>• Keloids—unsightly red and raised scars<br>• Skin irregularities<br>• Abnormal body contour<br>• Nerve damage<br>• Skin irregularities<br>• Skin death (necrosis)<br>• Infection<br>• Perforation of bowel or abdominal wall<br>• Slow healing—particularly if the patient is a smoker |
| **Duration of results** | Long-lasting |

# LARGE-VOLUME LIPOSUCTION
*Total body liposuction*

## What is large-volume liposuction?

**Large volume liposuction is a different operation than conventional liposuction. It involves surgery in at least five body areas, all at once, whereas conventional liposuction treats only localized areas. Large-volume liposuction can take up to 6 in (15 cm) off your waist, and sculpts your body. Some patients only need localized lipo to remove fat in the places where it stubbornly refuses to shift through diet or exercise, but for patients who are very overweight and need a whole-body size reduction, this may be the right procedure.**

### WHY HAVE LARGE-VOLUME LIPO?

Large-volume liposuction is defined as the removal of more than 10 pints (5 liters) total volume of fat and other fluids from the patient by suction using a long, fine, hollow metal tube, or cannula. Large-volume liposuction is usually used to treat patients who are 30–40 lb (15–20 kg) overweight, who need a significant reduction in fat and body measurements. Liposuction surgery can treat areas of excess fat in the stomach, buttocks, hips, waist, hips, thighs, calves, ankles, breasts, back, arms, and neck.

Due to the amount of fat being removed, the operation takes longer than conventional body-sculpting liposuction. Nearly all large-volume lipo operations are performed under general anesthetic and most patients stay in the hospital for at least one night after surgery.

Large-volume liposuction is a major operation, and certain criteria must be adhered to by the medical team to ensure that serious complications or even death do not occur.

**These criteria are:**

- The liposuction surgeon must be properly trained and educated in liposuction surgery and have a thorough understanding of the physiological changes that occur with conventional lipo and large-volume lipo.
- The anesthetist working with the liposuction surgeon also must be trained and have a complete understanding of the physiology associated with infusion and removal of large volumes of fluids.

- The facility where the liposuction operation is performed must be completely equipped to deal with any problem or complication that may occur during or after the procedure. The facility should be certified and accredited by a nationally recognized surgery accreditation body.
- The support staff working in the operating room and recovery room should be thoroughly trained and familiar with the liposuction procedure, as well as the care of the patient.
- The patient must be an appropriate candidate for the procedure.

Large-volume liposuction can improve a person's overall medical condition by reducing their cholesterol count and insulin requirements. It may also lower the risk or prevent the development of adult-onset diabetes in some patients. By significantly reducing your total body fat, either by liposuction or by other means of fat loss, you can potentially reduce the risk of heart disease, though the risks of undergoing the liposuction operation should be weighed against this.

There are limits to how much fat can safely be removed in one procedure, and you might need to undergo more than one to achieve the optimal result. Once you have liposuction, the fat cells are gone forever. However, it is still important to start or maintain a healthy lifestyle and balanced diet, because if you overeat, you will still gain weight. The weight will simply appear in areas of the body that still retain fat cells.

## Am I a candidate for a large-volume liposuction?

The best candidates for large-volume liposuction are in good physical and emotional health and have realistic expectations of what surgery can accomplish. Liposuction can provide a significant improvement, but it is unlikely to achieve perfection.

### Before undergoing large-volume liposuction, ask yourself:
- Have I tried diet and exercise?
- Am I overweight, but have maintained a stable weight for many years?
- Am I in generally good health?
- Is my excess fat in specific areas?
- Does my skin have reasonably good elasticity?

### WHAT TO EXPECT FROM A CONSULTATION WITH A LIPOSUCTION SURGEON

A full consultation with a board-certified, reputable surgeon who has experience of performing large-volume liposuction procedures will determine whether you are a suitable candidate. Your surgeon will estimate the amount of fat that should be removed from each area to achieve your desired body shape.

# The basic procedure

Large-volume liposuction is a major operation and can take between 1 and 2 hours. You will be given a general anesthetic and you may need to stay in hospital overnight afterward. The procedure is the same as for conventional liposuction (see pages 132 to 139) but carried out on a large scale or on more than one area of the body.

## Recovery and healing

Large-volume liposuction recovery times are normally longer than conventional liposuction recovery times. Large-volume liposuction is a major operation that requires general anesthetic. It is a much more serious operation than tumescent liposuction, which requires only local anesthetic. The recovery period is therefore longer than with other types of liposuction, and you may need to take several weeks off work to fully recover from the operation.

The first few days after surgery, you should rest as much as possible. You will likely be wearing a compression garment, a tight-fitting piece of surgical clothing that helps to heal the body and reduce swelling.

During the first 48 hours after surgery, patients experience varying degrees of swelling and bruising. The swelling persists longer. Bruising typically disappears within 7–10 days. Stitches are usually removed within 1 week of surgery. Avoid straining, bending over, and lifting during the early postoperative period.

When you wake up the results will be immediately obvious. The appearance of the treated areas will continue to improve once swelling subsides, and your unwanted fat will be gone forever, resulting in a slimmer, smoother body contour.

Other aspects of healing and recovery are the same as for conventional liposuction (see pages 132 to 139).

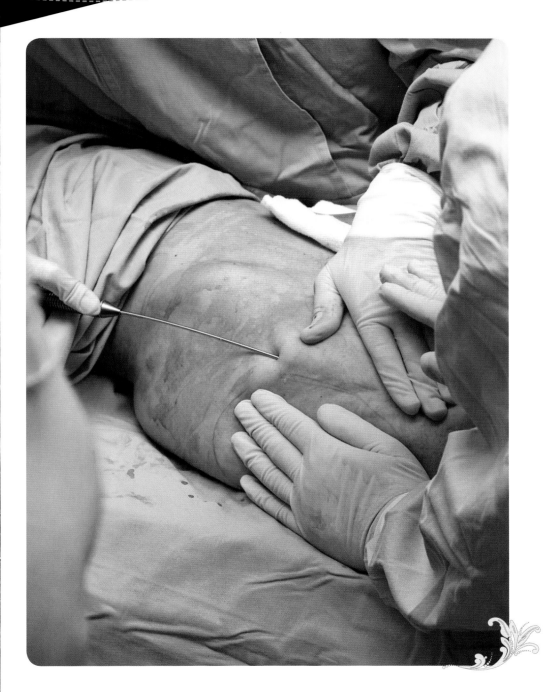

# TUMMY TUCK
## *Abdominoplasty*

### WHY HAVE A TUMMY TUCK?

Tummy tuck surgery is a procedure used to give a tighter, flatter stomach and reduce the appearance of stretch marks on the lower abdomen. This type of surgery is performed on patients who have skin and abdominal wall slackness after pregnancy or significant weight loss.

## *What is a tummy tuck?*

**Abdominoplasty offers a solution by flattening the slack skin and tightening the muscles of the relaxed tummy wall and, if needed, excess subcutaneous fatty tissue can be removed as well. It not only results in a better appearance, but it also stops the slackening process of the abdominal wall. The results can be long-lasting, especially if you exercise, eat a healthy diet, and maintain a healthy weight after your operation.**

## *There are three types of tummy tuck:*

### STANDARD TUMMY TUCK

The surgeon makes cuts into your abdomen and above your bikini line. Your belly button is cut from the surrounding skin. Stretched or torn muscles are pulled together and stitched into place and excess fat is removed. Your skin is then pulled down and the excess trimmed off. Your belly button will then be repositioned to fit the new shape of your tummy. The cuts are closed with stitches and your lower abdomen is firmly strapped with bandages. You will have a scar around your belly button and a long, curved scar along your bikini line, which can usually sit below the line of your underwear.

### MINI TUMMY TUCK

Only the skin and fat below your belly button are removed, leaving a long, curved scar along your bikini line.

### EXTENDED TUMMY TUCK

Excess skin and fat from your abdomen and your back is removed. You will have a scar around your belly button and a long curved scar along your bikini line and around your back.

# Am I a candidate for a tummy tuck procedure?

The ideal candidate for tummy tuck surgery is a patient in relatively good physical shape, who is unhappy with an excess of skin or fat in the abdominal area which is resistant to exercise. Often women who have been through pregnancy and childbirth have a laxity of underlying muscles, which makes it very difficult to achieve a flat and firm tummy again. This is because the skin and muscles have stretched beyond the point where they can naturally return to their normal location and shape.

Other ideal candidates for abdominoplasty are those who have lost a significant of weight and have excess sagging skin in the abdominal area. Older patients, who may have lost skin elasticity or have sagging skin due to the aging process, are also good candidates.

You must be prepared for the fact that abdominoplasty operations leave a permanent scar, normally across the full width of the bikini line. However, a good surgeon will ensure that the incision is made in such a way and in such a location that it can be easily hidden below your underwear.

**You should not consider surgery if:**
- You are a woman who is considering further pregnancies—the muscles pulled together and repaired during the tummy tuck procedure can separate again during pregnancy
- You are very overweight
- You are diabetic
- You are a smoker and/or have poor circulation
- You have visible scars from past abdominal surgeries and don't want further scarring on your body.

# Preparing for a tummy tuck procedure

**Your surgeon may ask you to:**
- Lose weight—you will get the optimum result if you are the correct weight for your height
- Stop taking the contraceptive pill six weeks before surgery—this reduces the risk of blood clotting
- Give up smoking
- Avoid taking aspirin, anti-inflammatory drugs, and herbal supplements.

Your surgeon may mark the operation site by drawing lines on your tummy, and with your consent may take photographs so that the results of your abdominoplasty before and after can be compared. You will then be prepared for theater, and you will be asked to wear compression stockings to help prevent blood clots. You will be measured for a support garment to wear after the operation to aid recovery.

## *The basic procedure*

Complete abdominoplasty usually takes 2–5 hours, depending on the extent of work required; partial abdominoplasty (a mini tummy tuck) may take 1–2 hours.

### 1. ANESTHESIA

The choices include intravenous sedation and general anesthetic. Your surgeon will recommend the best choice for you. If you have general anesthetic you will sleep through the operation. Depending on your medical history, your surgeon may use local anesthetic combined with a sedative to make you drowsy. You'll be awake but relaxed, and your abdominal region will be insensitive to pain, though you may feel a tugging sensation or some discomfort.

### 2. THE INCISIONS

**Full abdominoplasty:**

- A horizontal incision is made from hip to hip between the pubic area and navel. The shape and length of the incision depends on the degree of correction needed.
- Another incision is made to free the navel from the surrounding skin.
- The skin is detached from the abdominal wall to reveal the muscles and fascia to be tightened. The muscle fascia are tightened with sutures.
- The remaining skin and fat are tightened by removing the excess and closing the defect.

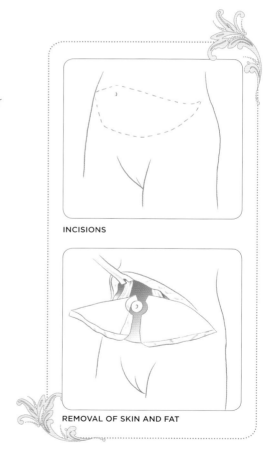

INCISIONS

REMOVAL OF SKIN AND FAT

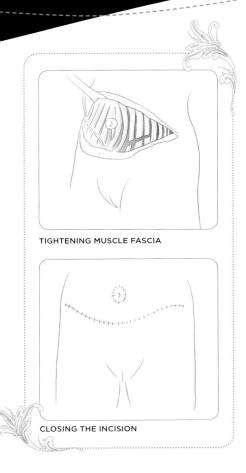

TIGHTENING MUSCLE FASCIA

CLOSING THE INCISION

**Opposite and above:**
**A full tummy tuck procedure**
**can take up to five hours**
**to perform.**

- The old belly button stalk is brought out through a new hole and sutured into place.
- Liposuction is often used to refine the transition zones of the abdominal sculpture.
- A dressing and sometimes a compression garment are applied and any excess fluid from the site is drained.

**Partial (mini) abdominoplasty:**
- A smaller incision is made.
- The skin and fat of the lower abdomen are detached in a more limited fashion from the muscle fascia. The skin is stretched down and excess skin removed.
- Sometimes the belly button stalk is divided from the muscle below and the belly button slid down lower on the abdominal wall.
- Sometimes a portion of the abdominal muscle fascia is tightened.
- Liposuction is often used to contour the transition zone.
- The flap is stitched back into place.

### 3. CLOSING THE INCISIONS

Sutures, skin adhesives, tapes, or clips are used to close the incisions.

### 4. THE RESULTS

Your tummy tuck will result in a flatter, firmer abdominal contour that is more proportionate with your body type and weight, and within a week or two you will be able to see your new, slimmer profile.

# Recovery and healing

Abdominoplasty recovery times vary depending on the extent of the tummy tuck operation, and the surgical techniques used. Abdominoplasty patients stay in hospital at least overnight and usually for a further two or three days. You will experience pain, but will be prescribed pain relief.

While you are still in the hospital, the catheter will usually be taken out during the first day. You may feel uncomfortable to begin with and have sudden urges to urinate, or have some difficulty emptying your bladder; this should pass within 24 hours. You will be wearing a compression garment (which should be changed after a week), which supports your abdomen and helps you to heal, and will probably feel a sensation of skin pulling and tenderness in the affected areas. These are common side effects, and will disappear in a couple of weeks. Don't strain or stretch the healing wound as this will increase swelling and slow your recovery. Continue wearing your support garment for at least 1 month.

Stitches in your skin are usually removed in 5–7 days. Deeper stitches are taken out two to three weeks after surgery. Ensure that you attend all follow-up exams with your doctor.

Full abdominoplasty recovery can take 3–6 months, and your scars will continue to fade after that time.

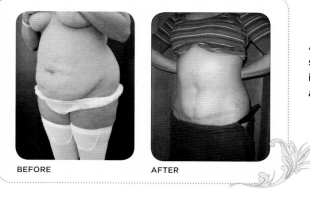

BEFORE      AFTER

**Abdominoplasty reduces stretch marks and results in a tighter, flatter appearance.**

# FACTS
## TUMMY TUCK SURGERY

| | |
|---|---|
| **Description** | A procedure used to give a tighter, flatter stomach and reduce the appearance of stretch marks on the lower abdomen. |
| **Length of surgery** | 2–5 hours |
| **In/outpatient** | Inpatient |
| **Anesthesia** | General |
| **Back to work in...** | 2–4 weeks |
| **Back to the gym in...** | 6 weeks |
| **Treatment frequency** | Once |
| **Risks** | • Considerable bruising—can take a month to clear<br>• Swelling—usually settles after a few months<br>• Scarring—will fade over the course of a year, but a permanent scar will remain<br>• Infection<br>• Hematoma<br>• Numbness—temporary or permanent<br>• Uneven contour<br>• Pigmentation changes<br>• Unfavorable scarring<br>• Fat necrosis<br>• Poor healing—more likely if you are a smoker<br>• Nerve damage<br>• Possibility of revision surgery<br>• Damage to internal organs<br>• Unusually red or raised scars (keloids)<br>• Pulmonary embolism |
| **Duration of results** | Long-lasting |

# BUTTOCK SURGERY
## Gluteoplasty

### WHY HAVE BUTTOCK SURGERY?

If you feel that your bottom could be shapelier or more curvaceous or that it is not in proportion with the rest of your body, then gluteoplasty, commonly known as buttock surgery, could be the solution for you.

## What is buttock surgery?

Buttock surgery comprises buttock implants or a buttock lift, or both. In 2008, 853 people in the U.S. opted for buttock or gluteal implants, according to the American Society of Plastic Surgeons. Of these, 87 percent were women who wanted either to emulate well-known female celebrities or to reverse the effects of aging.

## Am I a candidate for buttock surgery?

**You may be a suitable candidate if:**

- You are unhappy with the size and shape of your buttocks
- You have poor skin tone in the buttock area—characterized by loose or excess skin, stretch marks and cellulite
- You are physically and psychologically well and healthy
- You are over 18 years of age
- You are a non-smoker
- You have realistic expectations.

### WHAT TO EXPECT FROM A CONSULTATION WITH A BUTTOCK SURGEON

During this initial visit, be open about what you are looking to achieve through surgery. Discuss your goals and wishes, including how large you want your buttocks to be and how you would like them reshaped. The surgeon will also take a full medical history during your consultation to make sure you are healthy enough to undergo the buttock surgery.

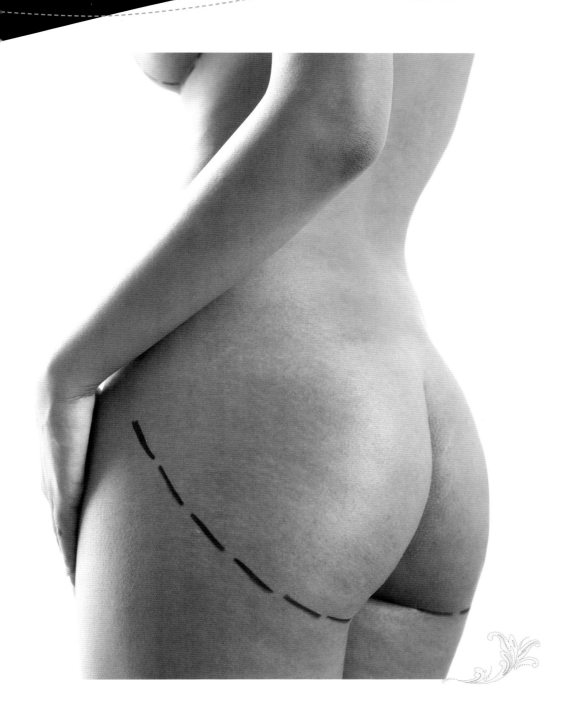

## Buttock surgery options

### BUTTOCK LIFT

A buttock lift is a surgical procedure to remove excess fat and loose skin in the buttock area, and may be combined with liposuction to further improve body contour. The procedure involves cutting the skin high up on the side of the thigh and buttocks, removing excess fat, and trimming away the excess skin. Liposuction and implants may also be used to create the desired result. The scars are strategically placed at the waistline or below to minimize their appearance in swimwear or underwear.

### BUTTOCK IMPLANTS

A fairly new development, the popularity of buttock implants has grown steadily, mainly because of the growing acceptance of cosmetic surgery procedures and changing fashions. Buttock implant surgery is now believed to have reached a tipping point, with more surgeons learning how to perform the surgery and increasing awareness among potential patients.

## The basic procedure: Buttock lift

### 1. ANESTHESIA

The buttock lift is normally carried out under a general anesthetic; sometimes an epidural may be used.

### 2. THE INCISIONS

The surgeon will make an incision across the top of the buttock, and depending on the extent of the operation, sometimes along the sides as well. Crescent-shaped sections of skin and fat are removed and the skin is pulled together.

### 3. THE SUTURES

The skin is pulled together over the new body contour, the incisions are sutured, and drains to remove blood or other fluids may be inserted.

### 4. THE RESULTS

The results of your buttock lift will initially be obscured by swelling, which may take 3–4 months to disappear. The final results will then begin to emerge.

# The basic procedure: Buttock implants

## 1. ANESTHESIA

The buttock implants are normally inserted under a general anesthetic, or local anesthetic with sedation.

## 2. THE INCISIONS

The surgeon makes an incision where the cheek meets the back of the thigh, or down the buttock crease. The doctor creates a pocket into which to insert the buttock implants, under or on top of the gluteus maximus muscle. Sometimes the operation is performed in combination with liposuction (see pages 132–139). After both buttocks have been operated on, the surgeon makes sure that the buttocks look symmetrical and natural.

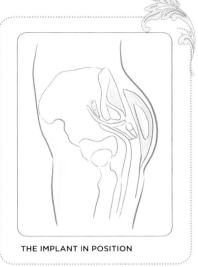

**THE IMPLANT IN POSITION**

## 3. THE SUTURES

The surgeon sutures the incisions with dissolvable stitches. A compression bandage is placed around the buttocks to help reduce discomfort and swelling.

## 4. THE RESULTS

The results of the operation can be seen immediately but the buttocks look more natural and become softer as the muscle stretches during the several months after surgery.

# Fat injections

Buttock implants can't help shape the lower part of the buttocks. However, fat injections can... The surgeon will remove fat from areas of the body where it is more plentiful (the flanks, hips, lower back, thighs, or abdomen) with liposuction. This excess fat is then purified and re-injected it into your backside.

Fat injections may also be used in other areas of the buttocks to sculpt, contour, and project the buttocks.

A full surgical procedure using only fat grafting is called a "Brazilian butt lift." In such cases, approximately 30 percent of the injected fat dissolves, meaning that the procedure may need to be repeated several months later.

# Recovery and healing

When you wake up after buttock implant surgery, you will feel tired, sore, and stiff, and will have swelling and bruising around your buttock area. You may be prescribed an antibiotic, pain medication, and an anti-inflammatory medication. You will wear a compression garment, which will be removed a few days after surgery.

During recovery, rest as much as possible, and drink plenty of fluids. You will be able to resume sedentary work within a few days to 1 week. Avoid physical exertion for several weeks. The stitches will come out within 1 week to 10 days, and swelling will gradually subside over several weeks. The results will then become apparent.

Swelling and bruising will be present for 10 to 14 days after a buttock lift, and discomfort and tightness in the buttock area is common for the first 24–48 hours. You will wear a supportive compression bandage over the area to help with the reduction of swelling and tightening of skin.

Most patients are back to work within a week or two after a buttock lift. Vigorous physical activity should be avoided for about 3–6 weeks. It is important to stay as mobile as possible during the buttock lift recovery time to promote good circulation and effective healing.

# FACTS
## BUTTOCK SURGERY

| | |
|---|---|
| **Description** | Improvement of the shape and appearance of the buttocks through implant, or lift, or both. |
| **Length of surgery** | 2 hours |
| **In/Outpatient** | Inpatient |
| **Anesthesia** | General or epidural |
| **Back to work in...** | A few days to 1 week |
| **Back to the gym in...** | 3–6 weeks |
| **Treatment frequency** | Once |
| **Risks** | • Swelling<br>• Bruising<br>• Tight feeling in the buttocks<br>• Numbness<br>• Pain<br>• Infection<br>• Blood clots<br>• Allergic reaction to the anesthetic<br>• Hematoma<br>• Seroma<br>• Skin necrosis (skin death)<br>• Unfavorable scarring<br>• Poor wound healing<br>• Asymmetry<br>• The implants may shift<br>• The implants may rupture |
| **Duration of results** | Long-lasting |

# THIGH LIFT
## Thigh reduction

## What is a thigh lift?

Thigh reduction surgery removes excess skin and fat from the inside and the outside of the upper thigh. The surgery leaves a long, noticeable scar. Thigh reduction improves the body contour in clothes, but the scars will be visible in underwear or swimwear.

### WHY HAVE A THIGH LIFT?

Thigh lift is a surgical procedure done to tighten sagging muscles and remove excess skin in the thigh area. Thigh lift surgery can be performed in conjunction with other procedures such as body lift.

## There are several types of thigh lift:

### INNER THIGH LIFT

This type of thigh lift helps people who have trouble eliminating excess fat from this area of the body through diet and exercise. It may also be used to treat reduced skin elasticity caused by the aging process or extreme weight loss. During an inner thigh lift, an incision is made at the junction of the thigh and pubic area. A wedge of skin, and possibly fat, is then removed and the skin is tightened to provide an improved leg contour and enhanced skin elasticity.

### BILATERAL THIGH LIFT

The bilateral thigh lift procedure is designed to tighten skin on the front and outside of the leg. During a bilateral thigh lift, the surgeon makes an incision at the top of the leg where the lower edge of a bikini bottom would be. A certain amount of skin is then removed before the surgeon pulls the remaining skin up and attaches it to the same area. It serves to tighten the skin along both sides of the leg. This procedure is especially helpful for those who have excess skin after an extreme weight loss.

### MEDIAL THIGH LIFT

A medial thigh lift reduces excess skin and fat on the upper portion of the inner thigh. It is designed for patients who are dissatisfied with the shape of their legs or who would like to remove excess skin after weight loss. An incision is made in the groin that goes to the back of the crease of the buttock. Skin is then lifted and excess skin and fat are removed to improve the shape of the leg and tighten the skin.

# Am I a candidate for thigh lift surgery?

**You may be a suitable candidate for thigh lift if:**

- You are bothered by sagging or drooping skin on the upper thigh
- You have lost a lot of weight and have excess skin
- Your weight is relatively stable
- You are physically and emotionally well and healthy
- You are a non-smoker
- You have realistic expectations of what thigh lift surgery can accomplish for you.

Thigh lift surgery is not a substitute for weight loss. Certain medical conditions and medications may affect whether you are a suitable candidate for thigh lift surgery. A cosmetic surgeon will be able to assess whether it is suitable for you.

## WHAT TO EXPECT FROM A CONSULTATION WITH A THIGH LIFT SURGEON

You'll be asked a number of questions about your health, lifestyle, and what you expect from the operation. Your surgeon will evaluate your general health and any pre-existing health conditions or risk factors, examine and measure your body, including taking detailed measurements, and may take photographs for your medical record. The surgeon will recommend the best type of thigh lift surgery for you.

## The basic procedure

### 1. ANESTHESIA
The choices include intravenous sedation and general anesthetic. Your surgeon will recommend the best choice for you.

### 2. THE INCISIONS
Incision patterns vary from case to case. However, they are normally placed in the groin, extending downward, and then traversing around the back of the thigh. The underlying tissue is reshaped and tightened, and the skin is reduced and re-draped over the new, smoother body contour. Another technique involves an incision only in the groin area. Your thigh lift surgeon will determine the appropriate option for you.

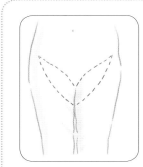
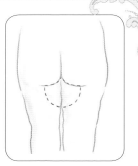

THIGH LIFT INCISIONS          ALTERNATIVE INCISIONS

### 3. THE SUTURES
Deep internal sutures within underlying tissues help to support the new contours. Sutures are used to close the skin incisions.

### 4. THE RESULTS
The smoother contouring is apparent almost immediately, although there will also be swelling and bruising.

## Recovery and healing

Dressings or bandages will be applied to your incisions, and you will be wrapped in an elastic bandage or a compression garment to minimize swelling and support your new contours as you heal. You may also have a drain fitted.

You will have some bruising and swelling, and tightness in the thighs.

The external stitches will be removed within 1 week, and the deeper sutures 2–3 weeks after. Recovery time is usually 1–2 weeks. You should be able to return to work after 2–3 weeks. Most swelling will disappear after about 3 weeks. You should avoid strenuous activity for about 1 month.

# FACTS
## THIGH LIFT SURGERY

| | |
|---|---|
| Description | A surgical procedure done to tighten sagging muscles and remove excess skin in the thigh area. |
| Length of surgery | 3 hours |
| In/outpatient | Outpatient or inpatient |
| Anesthesia | General |
| Back to work in... | 2–3 weeks |
| Back to the gym in... | 1 month |
| Treatment frequency | Once |
| Risks | • Bruising<br>• Swelling<br>• A tight feeling in the thighs<br>• Infection<br>• Blood clots<br>• Allergic reaction to the anesthetic<br>• Hematoma<br>• Seroma<br>• Unfavorable scarring<br>• Poor wound healing |
| Duration of results | Long-lasting |

# CALF IMPLANTS
## *Calf augmentation*

### WHY HAVE CALF IMPLANTS?

Calf augmentation creates cosmetic fullness in the lower leg. It corrects muscle imbalance as a result of both physical and congenital defects such as "skinny/chicken" legs, bow legs, club foot, or disproportionate calf development.

## *What is calf augmentation?*

Calf implants, made of soft, solid silicone, are placed in "pockets" overlying the existing muscles. Depending on the desired effect, one or two implants may be inserted. The appearance of the existing muscles in the calf area is thus made larger and more defined. Men typically undergo calf augmentation to emphasize bulk. Women undergo the procedure for a more proportionate appearance. The operation is carried out as an outpatient procedure, and takes about 1 hour.

## *Am I a candidate for calf augmentation surgery?*

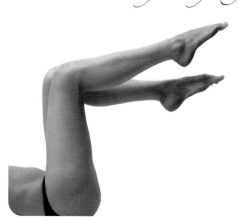

**You may be suitable if:**

- You are in good physical and psychological health
- You are unhappy with the size and shape of your calf area
- Exercise does not build muscle in your calf area
- You have realistic expectations for the surgery.

**A calf implant is placed just above the muscle.**

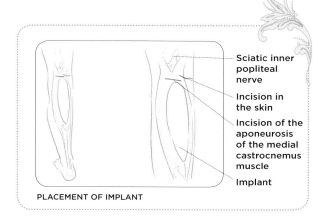

Sciatic inner popliteal nerve

Incision in the skin

Incision of the aponeurosis of the medial castrocnemus muscle

Implant

PLACEMENT OF IMPLANT

## *The basic procedure*

### 1. ANESTHESIA
You will be given either general or local anesthetic.

### 2. THE INCISIONS
An incision is made in the natural crease located at the back of the knee. A special instrument is used to create a pocket between the fascia (fibrous muscle covering) and the underlying muscle. This pocket is made just large enough for the implant to fit into securely and the implant is placed just above the muscle. The same procedure is performed on the other leg.

### 3. SUTURING
The surgeon carefully examines both legs to make sure they look symmetrical and natural. If so, stitches are used to close up the incisions.

### 4. THE RESULTS
The altered appearance of your calves will be immediately apparent, though it will be some months before the final results of your calf augmentation can be seen.

## *Preparing for calf augmentation surgery*

The calf-implant procedure does not affect muscle tone; therefore, you should speak with your surgeon about how to tone and firm the muscle beneath the skin before and after the procedure.

You also should make arrangements ahead of time for someone to drive you to and from the procedure and to assist you with your daily activities during your recovery period.

# Recovery and healing

When you come round after calf augmentation surgery, your legs will be elevated over a few pillows and you will be wearing a compression garment that covers your knees and calves. There will be some swelling, bruising, and numbness, which will subside. You will be advised to keep moving your toes and feet to ensure good circulation. You may feel muscle cramps, pressure, and tightness in your calves. Antibiotics and pain medication may be prescribed for you.

Calf augmentation recovery times vary from patient to patient. You should be able to walk normally after 2–3 weeks, and may return to work at this time. Avoid vigorous sporting activities for up to 2 months after calf augmentation surgery. You may return to full physical activities in 4–6 weeks.

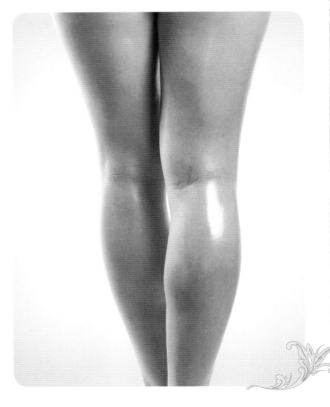

# FACTS
## CALF AUGMENTATION SURGERY

| | |
|---|---|
| **Description** | A surgical procedure to create cosmetic fullness in the lower leg. |
| **Length of surgery** | 1 hour |
| **In/Outpatient** | Outpatient |
| **Anesthesia** | General or local |
| **Back to work in...** | 2–3 weeks |
| **Back to the gym in...** | 4–6 weeks |
| **Treatment frequency** | Once |
| **Risks** | • Swelling<br>• Bruising<br>• Numbness<br>• Muscle cramps<br>• Infection<br>• Bleeding<br>• Blood clots<br>• Nerve and/or muscle damage<br>• Allergic reaction to the anesthetic<br>• Hematoma<br>• Seroma<br>• Unfavorable scarring<br>• Implant slippage<br>• Poor wound healing<br>• Asymmetry |
| **Duration of results** | Permanent |

# UPPER AND LOWER ARM LIFT
## *Brachioplasty*

## What is an upper and lower arm lift?

Due to the natural aging process, skin on the upper arms may become loose and flabby with a loss of elasticity. Substantial weight loss may be another cause of excess loose skin in this area. Often, such sagging skin cannot be improved by regular exercise or healthy diet alone, and may cause embarrassment, resulting in long-sleeved tops being worn to cover up the problem area. An arm lift can help to restore the area by giving a firmer and more youthful appearance.

### WHY HAVE AN ARM LIFT?

An arm lift, for the upper and lower regions of the arm, is a surgical procedure that reshapes the arm to reduce excess sagging skin, remove fat, and smooth and tighten the overall appearance.

## Am I a candidate for upper and lower arm lift surgery?

You may be a suitable candidate if:

- You have excess or loose and sagging upper and lower arm skin
- Your upper and lower arms have localized fat deposits
- Diet and exercise have not worked
- You have realistic expectations for the outcome of surgery.

You may not be suitable if you have had:

- A mastectomy or other operation on the armpit lymph node
- Infections in the sweat glands under the arm
- Healing problems after previous operations or procedures
- Keloid scarring.

You will not be suitable if you are more than 15 percent over your ideal body weight.

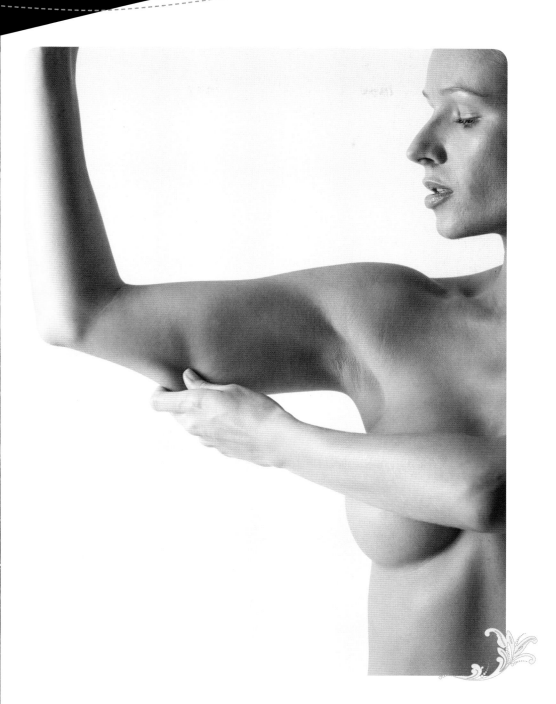

## The basic procedure

### 1. ANESTHETIC
Local anesthetic, local anesthetic with sedation, or general anesthetic is administered. The surgeon will decide what is most appropriate in your case.

### 2. THE INCISIONS
Incisions are made on the inside of the arm or on the back of the arm, from the underarm to just above the elbow and the under-surface of the arm, usually in a zigzag line. The skin is removed, then excess fat is excised or treated with liposuction. The remaining skin is stretched over the arm and sutured into place. A drain may be used at the site of the incision.

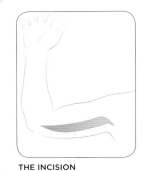

THE INCISION

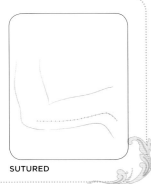

SUTURED

### 3. THE SUTURES
The incisions are closed with absorbable or removable sutures, and then bandaged.

### 4. THE RESULTS
The smoother, tighter contours of your arms will be apparent almost immediately, though there will be some swelling and bruising. It may take up to 2 years to see the final results.

## Recovery and healing

You can go home a day or so after your brachioplasty. Upper and lower arm lift recovery times vary from 1–2 weeks. Swelling and redness usually disappear after a month, and numbness may last for a few months. Use prescribed painkillers as required. Any drains and stitches are removed after 5–10 days and you will need to wear a surgical stocking for 3–4 weeks.

# FACTS
## ARM LIFT SURGERY

| | |
|---|---|
| **Description** | A surgical procedure that reshapes the arm to reduce excess sagging skin, remove fat, and smooth and tighten the overall appearance. |
| **Length of surgery** | 2 hours |
| **In/outpatient** | Outpatient |
| **Anesthesia** | Local or general |
| **Back to work in...** | 2 weeks |
| **Back to the gym in...** | 4–6 weeks |
| **Treatment frequency** | Once |
| **Risks** | • Bruising<br>• Swelling<br>• Redness<br>• Numbness<br>• Infection<br>• Blood clots<br>• Seroma<br>• Hematoma<br>• Excessive scarring<br>• Allergic reaction to the anesthetic |
| **Duration of results** | Long-lasting |

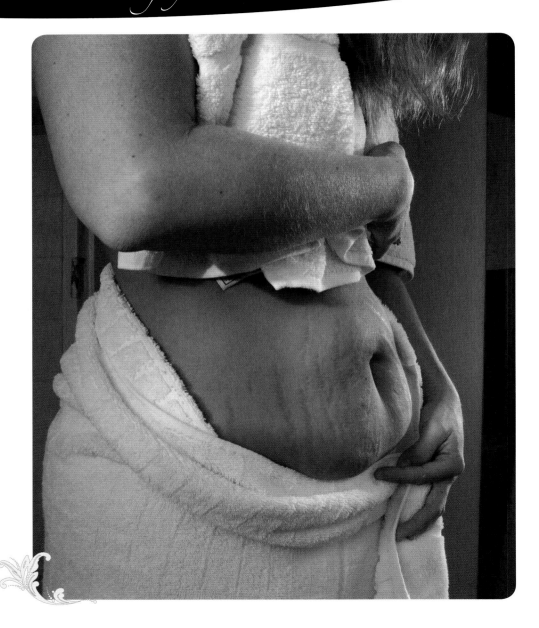

Weight-loss (bariatric) surgery refers to various procedures that are performed to treat obesity by modifying the gastrointestinal tract to affect nutrient intake and/or absorption when the patient eats. According to the American Society for Metabolic and Bariatric Surgery, an estimated 205,000 people with severe obesity had bariatric surgery in 2007 in the U.S. Patients who chose to lose weight through bariatric surgery accept a lifetime of changes—eating habits, lifestyle adjustments, and medical considerations.

Patients who have undergone bariatric surgery may typically experience dramatic weight loss, which can be maintained for up to 10 years after surgery. However, it can be very discouraging to achieve weight loss, yet still have to contend with excess skin that keeps you from wearing the clothes you'd like. Excess skin can also cause daily discomfort in the form of rashes and, possibly, skin infections. Post-weight loss cosmetic surgery can be an excellent solution for anyone who would like to have loose, excess skin removed from their body. Body contouring procedures can help you achieve the figure you desire after weight-loss surgery, post pregnancy, or following weight loss achieved through diet and exercise.

Such post-bariatric procedures include:

### FACE AND NECK LIFT
After dramatic weight loss, the facial skin can become loose and saggy, resulting in drooping cheeks and jowls, a loose and sagging neck area, and the loss of a defined jawline. A face and neck lift raises the cheek pads, corrects the jowls, and removes the loose and sagging skin. (See pages 44 and 74.)

### ARM LIFT (BRACHIOPLASTY)
As you age, the upper arm skin can become loose and flabby, which can be accentuated after significant weight loss. An arm lift can remove the excess skin and fat deposits, giving the upper arms a more tightened and defined contour. (See page 172.)

### BREAST LIFT (MASTOPEXY)
After dramatic weight loss, the breasts can sag and droop as the skin loses elasticity and fat is lost. A breast lift raises and firms sagging, flat breasts, sometimes also using breast implants to improve the shape and size of the breasts. (See page 114.)

## MEDIAL THIGH LIFT

A thigh lift tightens and improves the look of the skin of the inner thighs after weight loss. (See page 164.)

## TUMMY TUCK

Also known as abdominoplasty, a tummy tuck removes excess fat and skin, and in most cases restores weakened or separated muscles to create an abdominal profile that is smoother and firmer. (See page 152.)

## PANNICULECTOMY

This post-bariatric surgery removes the hanging pannus ("apron" of skin) from the lower abdomen below the belly button. A panniculectomy is often performed on patients who have lost a lot of weight but who still experience back problems, the breakdown of skin, rashes, ulcers, or other skin disorders that may make walking, standing, or even sitting extremely difficult. During the operation, the pannus is surgically excised. The surgeon makes two incisions on the lower abdomen, one horizontal and one vertical, to create an inverted "T" shape. A large, triangular-shaped area of loose skin and excess fat is carefully removed, and the remaining tissue is then attached to the anterior abdominal wall and to itself. Abdominoplasty can be performed alongside the panniculectomy to help tighten the stomach muscles.

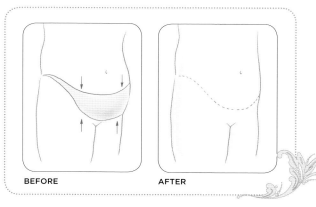

BEFORE          AFTER

**Panniculectomy removes the hanging "apron" of skin from the lower abdomen below the belly button.**

## LOWER BODY LIFT (BELT LIPECTOMY)

When an individual is overweight, the fat is normally deposited around their lower trunk area including the abdomen, back, buttocks, and outer and inner thighs. After losing a lot of weight, excess fat and skin remain in these areas. A lower body lift corrects the sagging skin of the abdomen, outer thighs, buttocks, hips, and waist in one procedure. Excess skin and fat are surgically removed and the remaining tissue and skin lifted, which results in a tighter and smoother appearance of the buttock and thigh areas. A tummy tuck and liposuction may also be performed at the same time. The belt lipectomy surgery involves long cuts, which result in long scars. The length of the cuts and the resulting scars depends on how much excess skin needs to be removed. The surgeon will usually try to position the incisions so that they can be hidden beneath underwear.

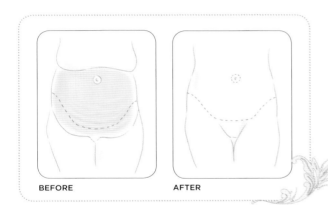

BEFORE          AFTER

**A lower body lift corrects the sagging skin of the abdomen, outer thighs, buttocks, hips, and waist all in one procedure.**

Before you decide to undergo a procedure, your weight should be stable. If you continue to lose weight, sagging "pockets" will develop. If you rapidly regain the weight, you will traumatically stress your already weakened and thinned skin, causing further stress to the skin, visible stretch marks, and wide scars. If you had weight reduction surgery, your cosmetic surgeon will work closely with your physician to determine when it is appropriate for you to begin body contouring.

**Good candidates are:**

- Adults of any age whose weight loss has been achieved and stabilized
- Healthy adults who do not have any medical conditions that might impair healing or increase the risks of surgery
- Non-smokers
- Individuals with a positive outlook and realistic expectations
- Individuals who can demonstrate a commitment to proper nutrition and fitness.

## WHAT TO EXPECT DURING A CONSULTATION FOR POST WEIGHT-LOSS SURGERY

Expect to be asked a number of questions by the surgeon about your health, lifestyle, and expectations, as well as your reasons for wanting the surgery. You will also discuss the various surgical options available. As with any surgery, you'll discuss your medical history, the risks involved in the surgery, and the surgeon will likely take photographs for your medical records.

## Is post weight-loss surgery for me?

Not everyone who achieves great weight loss or undergoes weight loss surgery will require subsequent cosmetic surgery. Before you lose all your weight, you can't really be sure whether you'll need cosmetic surgery afterward. Although there are no guarantees, here are some factors that affect whether you'll need post-weight loss cosmetic surgery:

**Your age:** People who are younger have more elasticity in their skin, and their skin will snap back more easily and much faster.

**How much weight you have to lose:** The more overweight you are, the more your skin is stretched, and the more likely you are to need cosmetic surgery.

**Where you carry your weight:** If the majority of your weight is concentrated in one area, such as your abdomen, rather than all over your body, then your chances of needing cosmetic surgery are increased.

**How many times you've gained and lost weight in your lifetime:** Your skin is like a balloon that goes up and down. Repeated stretching and shrinking cause the skin to lose elasticity over time.

**Whether you smoke:** Smoking breaks down collagen, a major component of skin and other structural components of the body. Smokers develop more loose and lax skin than non-smokers.

**Sun exposure and damage:** If your skin has suffered considerable sun exposure and damage your skin could be less elastic.

**Genetics:** Some skin types have more elasticity than others.

# Recovery and healing

Body contouring can require several days' hospitalization, up to six weeks off work, and it might take a year for the scars to heal. Recovery times vary from a couple of weeks to several weeks, depending on the extent of the surgery and the healing abilities of the individual patient. If multiple procedures are required then they are usually spread over several months.

After the body contouring procedure is complete, dressings or bandages will be applied to the incisions. A small, thin tube may be temporarily placed under the skin to drain any excess blood or fluid that may collect. As with all cosmetic surgery procedures, good results are generally expected, however there is no guarantee. In some circumstances, it may not be possible to achieve optimal results with a single surgical procedure and another operation may be necessary.

The results of a body contouring following extensive weight loss are visible almost immediately. However, it may take as long as 1–2 years or more for the final results to be evident. It is important to accept that visible scars from body contouring cosmetic surgery will remain, but the overall results are long-lasting, provided that you maintain a stable weight and general fitness.

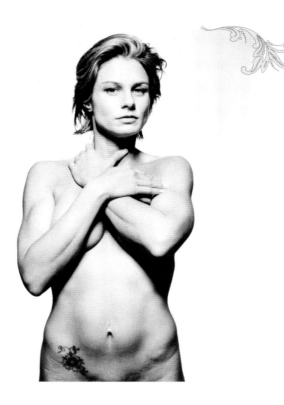

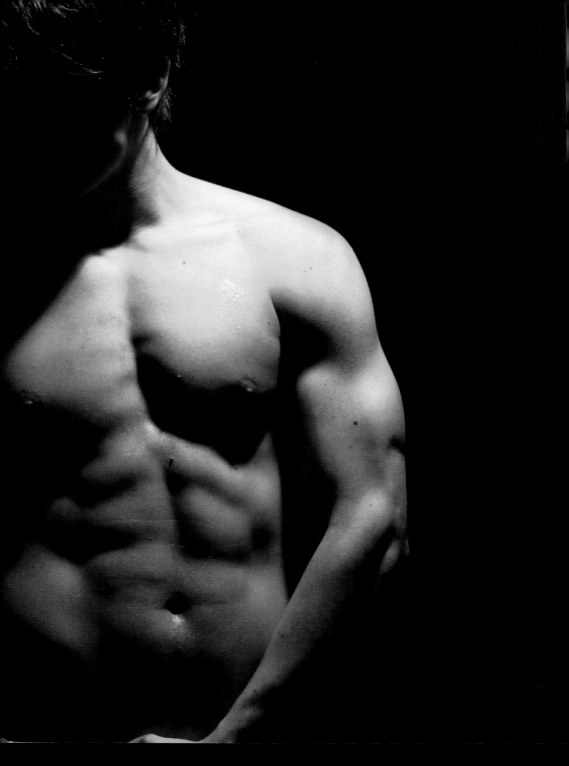

# CHAPTER FIVE
# MALE COSMETIC SURGERY

# MALE COSMETIC SURGERY
*An overview*

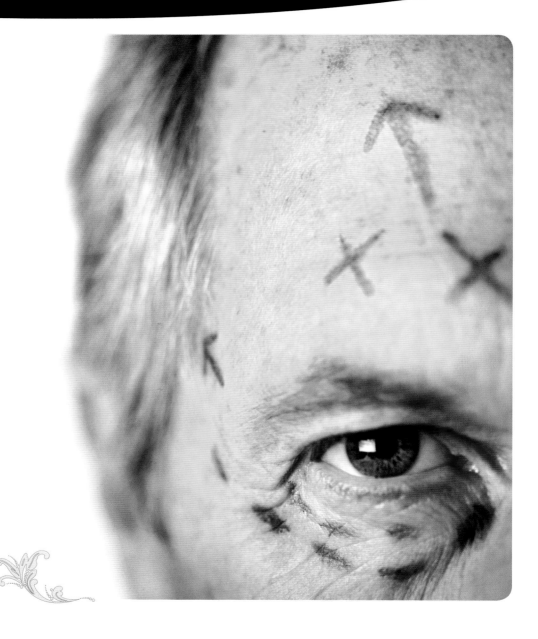

Cosmetic surgery is chosen by men who want to reverse the effects of the aging process or attain a new physique that might not be achieved through exercise and a healthy diet. Male cosmetic surgery procedures can give men bigger chests, trimmer waists, fewer wrinkles, more hair, and increased overall body confidence.

The following chapter explores the most popular procedures in more detail. These include:

- Pectoral enhancement
- Hair restoration
- Male breast reduction
- Male tummy tuck
- Male facelift
- Male nose surgery
- Male liposuction.

Women still form the majority of patients undergoing cosmetic surgery; however, with the shift in public opinion about cosmetic surgery, more and more men each year are now looking to the many procedures available to them in order to put physical "wrongs" right.

# PECTORAL ENHANCEMENT
*Chest implants*

## WHY HAVE PECTORAL IMPLANTS?

Pectoral enlargement is a cosmetic procedure in which implants made of solid silicone are inserted into the chest to increase its size and shape. This procedure is usually performed on men who have underdeveloped chest muscles, either because of a resistance to the effects of exercise or as the result of a growth defect or injury. Pectoral implants can create a larger, natural-looking chest area.

## *What is pectoral enhancement?*

**Some men work out extensively but still cannot develop the pectoral muscles they desire. Pectoral implants can give a defined outline to the chest and the appearance of high, firm pectoral muscles, as if the patient had been working out. The implants are made of solid silicone and, unlike female breast implants, pectoral implants do not carry the risk of rupturing and/or leaking. During the procedure, the implant is placed directly beneath the upper pectoral muscle.**

Pectoral implants can help build self-confidence in men who are embarrassed by their appearance. In the hands of a skilled surgeon, the result is a naturally muscular and "bulked-up" appearance, with a more well-proportioned torso. Pectoral implants are made in a number of sizes and shapes that mimic a well-developed pectoral muscle, and can also be custom-made.

Although most men have chest implants to obtain a more aesthetically pleasing, masculine appearance, some men with defects of the ribcage or chest muscles may have them to balance an asymmetrical or malformed chest. Implants will normally need to be custom-made in these cases and would require a specialist surgeon.

Men who have gynecomastia, the development of enlarged male breasts, may also have pectoral enlargement surgery after undergoing liposuction and removal of glandular breast tissue as part of a male breast reduction operation.

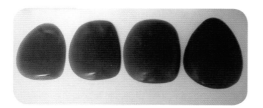

**Pectoral implants**

# Am I a candidate for pectoral enlargement?

This surgery can be performed at any age, and the best subjects are healthy, emotionally stable men who have skin with good elasticity that will readily adapt to the new contours. You must also have realistic expectations for the outcome.

**If any of the following apply to you, you may not be a good candidate:**

- You are asthmatic
- You have high blood pressure (hypertension)
- You use recreational drugs
- You drink excessively
- You smoke.

You must tell your surgeon about all the medications that you take, including vitamin and mineral supplements and herbal products.

## WHAT CAN I EXPECT FROM A CONSULTATION WITH A PECTORAL ENHANCEMENT SURGEON?

At the initial consultation, you should discuss exactly what you expect from the procedure and how you would like to look afterward. Your surgeon should tell you exactly what will be involved in the chest implant procedure and discuss any side effects, potential complications, and the recovery process. A full medical history should be taken to make sure that there are no reasons why you shouldn't have chest implants. You will then be asked to read information about the chest implant procedure and sign a consent form, which means that you have understood the potential benefits and risks. Photographs may also be taken for a "before and after" comparison at a later date.

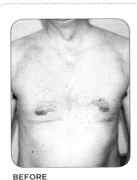

BEFORE

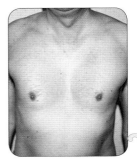

AFTER

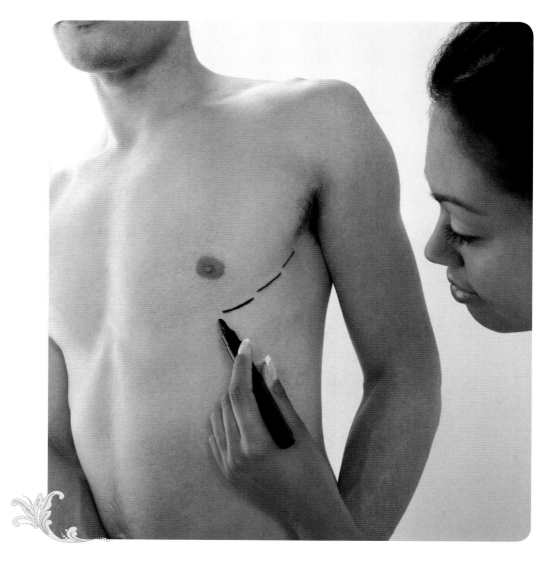

# The basic procedure

## 1. ANESTHESIA

Pectoral implant operations are usually carried out under general anesthetic, though sometimes your doctor will use local anesthetic and intravenous sedation, which will make you very drowsy. Your surgeon will recommend the best choice for you. It is possible to have a pectoral enhancement as day surgery, though you will normally need to stay in hospital overnight. The length of the procedure varies according to the technique used, the placement of the implants, the patient's anatomy, and the type of anesthesia used.

## 2. THE INCISIONS AND IMPLANTS

The surgeon will make a small incision in the armpit, and a small pocket under the pectoral muscle. Once the pocket is created, the implant is sculpted to the right size. The implant is inserted into the pocket and secured with a few small, dissolving sutures, using an endoscope—a thin tube with a tiny camera on the end. This method reduces incision size as well as bleeding, though non-endoscopic methods are sometimes preferred.

## 3. THE SUTURES

The incisions are then sutured and a dressing is applied to protect the incisions and reduce swelling. The implants are held in place by the overlying chest muscle or by sutures that are temporarily visible through the skin.

## 4. THE RESULTS

The results of pectoral surgery are immediately visible. Over time post-surgical swelling will subside and resolve, and incision lines will gradually refine in appearance. Someone will need to drive you home, and you may need assistance over the next couple of days.

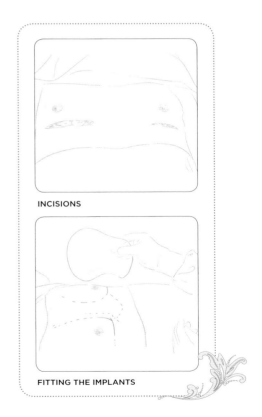

INCISIONS

FITTING THE IMPLANTS

**The process of pectoral enlargement is similar to breast enlargement.**

# Recovery and healing

Recovery times vary from patient to patient. You will feel some discomfort after chest implant surgery—this will last from a few days to several weeks and can be controlled by prescription medication. It is also quite common to experience a little numbness from bruised nerves in and around your chest area. Most of this should pass over time, as you heal.

You will usually be allowed to go home the day of your surgery. Your dressing and sutures will be removed in a few days. After a month, the scars usually fade and become barely perceptible.

You will need to wear a compression garment continuously for 1–2 weeks after surgery, and at night for a few weeks after that. The worst of your swelling will go down in the first few weeks but it may be 3 months or more before the final results of your surgery become apparent.

Your surgeon will also advise you to rest and sleep in an elevated position and apply cold compresses to reduce swelling. The sutures will dissolve naturally so do not need to be removed. Try to rest as much as possible, as your recovery will be much quicker if you do. Your surgeon will probably recommend that you walk around as soon as possible after surgery to help reduce swelling and lower the chances of blood clots forming in the legs, which can be extremely dangerous.

Drink plenty of fluids, and be sure to take your prescribed medications. Keep dry—avoid getting water on your wounds for a week. You will be instructed not to lift your arms after surgery. After the dressings are removed you may follow a gentle exercise program to improve mobility in your arms. This allows the pectoral implants to settle into the fascia pockets that surround the muscle.

If decide that you want your chest implants taken out, removal is relatively simple. This can be performed through the same incision and recovery is usually quicker than from the original surgery.

# FACTS
## PECTORAL ENHANCEMENT

| | |
|---|---|
| **Description** | A cosmetic procedure in which implants made of solid silicone are inserted into the chest to increase its size and shape. |
| **Length of surgery** | 1–2 hours |
| **In/outpatient** | Outpatient or inpatient |
| **Anesthesia** | General or local with sedative |
| **Back to work in...** | 1 week |
| **Back to the gym in...** | 1 month |
| **Treatment frequency** | Once |
| **Risks** | • Swelling, tenderness, numbness, and bruising<br>• Unfavorable scarring<br>• Hematoma<br>• Blood clots<br>• Infection<br>• Poor wound healing<br>• Numbness, which may be temporary or permanent<br>• Displacement of implants<br>• Breast contour and shape irregularities<br>• Skin discoloration, permanent pigmentation changes, swelling, and bruising<br>• Damage to skin or internal organs<br>• Breast asymmetry<br>• Fat necrosis<br>• Seroma<br>• Deep vein thrombosis, cardiac and pulmonary complications |
| **Duration of results** | Permanent |

# HAIR RESTORATION
*Hair transplantation*

## What is hair restoration?

**Male hair loss is caused by increased sensitivity to male sex hormones (androgens) in certain parts of the scalp, and is hereditary. The hormones make the hair follicles shrink until they become so small that they cannot replace lost hairs. Hair restoration is a surgical procedure in which hairs are taken from an area of the scalp resistant to baldness (usually the sides and the back of the head) and grafted to the bald area.**

### WHY HAVE HAIR RESTORATION?

With half the men in the United States suffering from hair loss by age 50, hair transplants have become the number one cosmetic procedure for men in the United States. Many women also suffer from thinning hair or patterns of baldness. Although hair-loss treatments do not work for everyone, hair transplants do offer permanent hair restoration for most patients. The goal is to give the natural-looking appearance of healthy hair.

Hair transplant surgery is a method of hair distribution. A hair transplant procedure always begins with your own healthy donor hair, located on the sides or the back of the head. This hair here is naturally resistant to balding. Most men with standard male pattern baldness will have a healthy donor area with plenty of viable hairs for the hair transplant surgery. However, if your hair loss is not hereditary and is caused by other conditions such as stress or medication, you will need to consult a dermatologist before considering a hair restoration procedure.

Different hair transplant clinics use different methods and technology to achieve results, and all require a skilled and experienced hair transplant surgeon. A successful hair transplant surgery will make the whole new head of hair appear natural, while maximizing hair growth and minimizing scalp trauma and scarring.

Surgical hair restoration begins with an evaluation of the donor area, located at the back and sides of the head. The hair restoration surgeon will select donor hairs from this area that are genetically programmed not to shed and are the most resistant to balding, making them the ideal hair for hair restoration. Only a trained specialist can judge whether you have the sufficient hair density needed for successful hair transplant surgery.

# Hair restoration techniques

## FOLLICULAR UNIT GRAFTING

In follicular unit hair transplantations, a small section of tissue with hairs is removed from the donor area and prepared for surgery under intense magnification. Follicular units grow in groups of one to four hairs. The hair transplant surgeon can graft different numbers of hairs and follicles including micrografts (one or two hairs), slit grafts (four to 10 hairs), and strip grafts (30 to 40 hairs).

The hair transplant surgeon places these follicular units at precise but varied angles in the frontal hair zone to create a soft, natural-looking hairline. Larger follicular units are placed behind the hairline, giving density and volume to the larger balding areas. Micrografts reproduce exactly how hair grows in nature and the hairs are transplanted in suitable areas, i.e. certain groups of hair and tissue are best suited to the hairline, others to the crown of the head. These tissue and hair groupings become embedded into the recipient site and will blend with the existing hair.

## FLAP SURGERY

There are also more extensive kinds of hair replacement surgery that can produce dramatic results in a much shorter time. A flap is an example of such surgery. This involves removing an area of scalp to be stitched to a balding spot yet maintaining the blood supply from the original donor site. Flap surgery on the scalp has been performed successfully for many years. This procedure is capable of quickly covering large areas of baldness and is customized for each individual patient. One flap can do the work of 350 or more punch grafts.

A section of bald scalp is cut out and a flap of hair-bearing skin is lifted off the surface while still attached at one end. The hair-bearing flap is brought into its new position and sewn into place, while remaining "tethered" to its original blood supply. As you heal, you'll notice that the scar is camouflaged by relocated hair.

In recent years, surgeons have made significant advances in flap techniques, combining flap surgery and scalp reduction for better coverage of the crown.

## SCALP REDUCTION

This technique is sometimes referred to as advancement flap surgery because sections of hair-bearing scalp are pulled forward or "advanced" to fill in a bald crown. Scalp reduction is for coverage of bald areas at the top and back of the head. It's not beneficial for coverage of the frontal hairline. After the scalp is injected with a local anesthetic, a segment of bald scalp is removed. The pattern of the section of removed scalp varies widely, depending on the patient's goals. If a large amount of coverage is needed, doctors commonly remove a segment of scalp in an inverted Y-shape.

The skin surrounding the cutout area is loosened and pulled, so that the sections of hair-bearing scalp can be brought together and stitched. It's likely that you'll feel a strong tugging, and occasional pain.

# Am I a candidate for hair restoration?

Men typically seek hair transplant surgery to correct hair loss resulting from genetics, aging, a traumatic injury, or certain medical conditions. The ideal hair transplant candidate must have existing healthy hair on the back or sides of the head. The candidate must also be prepared to undergo treatment in multiple sessions that can take several hours. The most important thing to consider when thinking about having hair restoration surgery is that you must have enough hair to be transplanted.

Patients over 30 normally make good hair transplant candidates, because people in their twenties have not yet developed a fixed pattern of hair loss. However, people in their early twenties who are starting to lose their hair and who have a family history of male pattern baldness can choose to have the procedure.

Hair loss affects individuals in different ways, but if you feel that your hair loss is negatively impacting on your self-esteem, your social life, your confidence and/or performance at work, and your self-assurance with the opposite sex, you may be a good candidate for hair restoration.

## WHAT TO EXPECT FROM A CONSULTATION WITH A HAIR RESTORATION SURGEON

Before committing to undergo hair replacement surgery, it is important to weigh up the benefits and risks of the procedure. Thanks to modern techniques, the benefits of hair replacement surgery are becoming greater and the risks fewer. During your consultation, your hair transplant surgeon will discuss the hair restoration procedure in detail with you, and talk to you about the side effects, risks, and possible complications so that you can make an informed decision about the hair transplant surgery. The surgeon will analyze the texture, density, and color of your donor hair, future hair loss projections, and your skin type to evaluate whether there is enough hair to transplant and if so, the number of grafts needed.

# The basic procedure

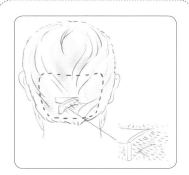

STRIP REMOVED FROM DONOR AREA

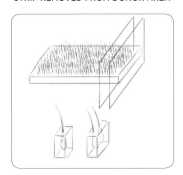

STRIP DIVIDED INTO FOLLICULAR
UNIT GRAFTS

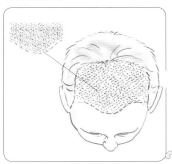

HAIR GRAFTS IMPLANTED INTO
INCISIONS IN HAIR LOSS AREA

## 1. ANESTHESIA

Local anesthesia is administered in the donor and recipient areas of the scalp. (The procedure is usually performed under local anesthetic, though general anesthetic may be used for more extensive hair transplant surgery.)

## 2. THE GRAFTS

Segments of the scalp (grafts) that contain hair from the denser donor area are removed using a sharp, carbon steel tube puncher or a scalpel and then attached to the recipient balding or thinning area. These grafts vary in size—mini-grafts contain up to four hairs; slit grafts that are inserted into slits in the scalp have up to 10 hairs; round-shaped punch grafts have up to ten hairs and strip grafts contain up to 40 hairs.

## 3. THE SUTURES

The donor skin site is stitched back together. There will be some scarring but it will be covered with hair.

## 4. THE RESULTS

Immediately following hair transplant surgery the recipient area is typically pink with scabs forming around the micro-incisions where the grafts were taken. These hundreds of tiny incisions will heal rapidly within 1 week to 10 days. The surgeon may prescribe medications to manage minimal discomfort, bruising, and swelling. The transplanted hair will often fall out within 6 weeks, but re-growth can be expected to occur within 3 months.

# Recovery and healing

You should feel well a day or two after your surgical hair restoration, although some numbness and mild soreness can be expected for several days following surgery. Normally it takes from 3–5 months before the transplanted hair follicles begin to grow new hair. The transplanted hair grows in very thin initially and gradually grows thicker and fuller over time. After one year a patient's transplanted hair will be fully mature and will continue to grow and the results should look entirely natural, even under close examination. This hair will continue to grow over your lifetime.

Approximately 24 hours after the surgery, small scabs will have formed on each of the grafts. This is normal, and they will usually be shed in about 7 to 10 days following hair replacement surgery. You should be able to gently wash your hair after 48 hours. Approximately 6 to 15 weeks after the hair transplant, the grafted hair should begin to grow at the normal hair-growth rate of $\frac{1}{2}$ in (1 cm) per month.

Hair replacement surgery is a complicated procedure that may require several transplant sessions over a period of one to two years before the desired result is achieved. However, this intricate process should produce new, natural-looking hair growth that will last a lifetime.

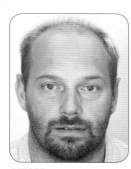

BEFORE

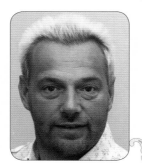

AFTER

# FACTS
## HAIR RESTORATION

| | |
|---|---|
| **Description** | A surgical procedure in which hairs are taken from an area of the scalp resistant to baldness and grafted to the bald area. |
| **Length of surgery** | Varies |
| **In/outpatient** | Outpatient (unless a large area is involved) |
| **Anesthesia** | Local |
| **Back to work in...** | 5–7 days |
| **Back to the gym in...** | 1–2 weeks |
| **Treatment frequency** | Once |
| **Risks** | • Small scabs that form over the graft areas<br>• Temporary thinning of pre-existing hair<br>• Mild pain and discomfort<br>• Numbness of the scalp—this is usually temporary and resolves in several months but can be permanent<br>• Bleeding<br>• Scarring<br>• Cysts<br>• Infection<br>• Transplanted hair may not survive the procedure |
| **Duration of results** | Long-lasting |

# MALE BREAST REDUCTION
## *Reduction mammoplasty*

## *What is male breast reduction?*

**Gynecomastia is a common condition that begins during puberty, in which firm, tender breast tissue grows under the nipples. It is usually caused by an imbalance of hormones, and normally disappears between the ages of 18 and 20 without treatment. In rare cases, gynecomastia may be caused by prescription drugs such as anabolic steroids, illegal drugs, tumors, or disease. In some cases, tests are needed. Whether you need tests depends on your age, your medical history, and the physical examination carried out by your cosmetic surgeon. Your doctor will ask you questions about your symptoms, such as how long you've had the breast tissue, and whether or not the area is tender.**

### WHY HAVE BREAST REDUCTION?

Male breast reduction removes excess fat and/or glandular tissue and skin and may be suitable for men who feel self-conscious about their "man breasts" (gynecomastia). It will create a flatter, firmer, and better-contoured chest.

Men who are self-conscious because they have overdeveloped or enlarged breast tissue (usually caused by being overweight, or having lost weight), or men who suffer from back and neck ache because their "breasts" are too heavy, can benefit from male breast reduction surgery. Some men and boys have fat on their chests that makes it look like they have breasts. This condition is called pseudogynecomastia.

Gynecomastia can cause emotional discomfort and affect a man's self-confidence. Some men will avoid taking their shirt off, avoid certain physical activities, and keep away from intimate situations to hide their condition. It may be present in one or both breasts. In severe cases, the weight of excess breast tissue may cause the breasts to sag and stretch the areola (the dark skin surrounding the nipple). In these cases the position and size of the areola can be surgically improved and excess skin may be reduced.

The final results of male breast reduction surgery are permanent in most cases; however, if your gynecomastia resulted from the use of prescription medications or from weight gain, you must be clean of these substances and/or lose weight in order to maintain your results.

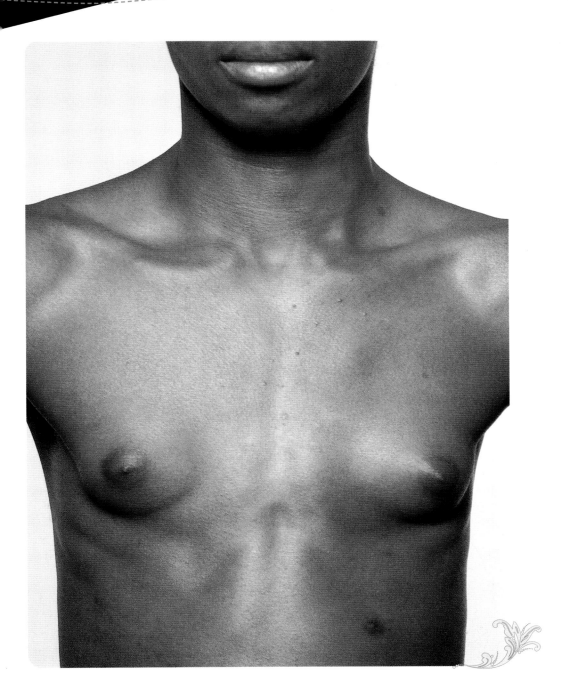

# Am I a candidate for male breast reduction surgery?

This surgery can be performed at any age, and the best subjects are healthy, emotionally stable men who have skin with good elasticity that will readily adapt to the new contours. You must also have realistic expectations for the outcome of the procedure.

Obese patients will be advised to try exercise and dieting to reduce the fat before having surgery.

### You may be a suitable candidate if:

- You are physically healthy and of normal, stable weight
- You have realistic expectations
- Your breasts have stopped developing
- You are unhappy with the size and appearance of your male breasts.

## WHAT TO EXPECT FROM A CONSULTATION WITH A MALE BREAST REDUCTION SURGEON

Your surgeon will examine your breasts and may take detailed measurements of their size and shape, the skin quality, and the placement of your nipples and areolas. Your surgeon will evaluate whether the excess tissue is fatty and/or glandular. Fatty tissue will be removed by liposuction, and glandular tissue is removed with a scalpel. There are various liposuction techniques that may be used; the technique most appropriate in your case will be discussed prior to your procedure.

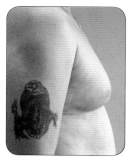

BEFORE

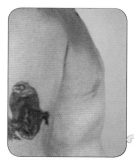

AFTER

**Male breast reduction creates a flatter, firmer, and better contoured chest.**

# The basic procedure

## 1. ANESTHESIA

Male breast reduction may be performed under local anesthetic with a sedative to make you relaxed. Alternatively, under a general anesthetic, you sleep through the whole operation. You will have agreed the most suitable choice beforehand with your surgeon.

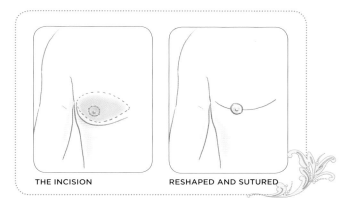

THE INCISION

RESHAPED AND SUTURED

## 2. THE INCISIONS AND TISSUE REMOVAL

Where the gynecomastia is primarily the result of excess fatty tissue, liposuction (usually ultrasound-assisted) techniques alone may be used. A small incision, less than ½ in (1 cm) long, is made around the edge of the dark skin that surrounds the nipple (the areola), or under the arm. A cannula is inserted and moved backward and forward in a controlled motion to loosen the excess fat, which is then removed from the body by vacuum. If glandular tissue or excess skin is to be removed to correct the gynecomastia, tissue may have to be removed with a scalpel. The incision is made in an inconspicuous location on the edge of the dark skin around the nipple (the areola) and the glandular tissue is removed. Major reductions may require larger incisions that result in longer scars. Excision is also necessary if the areola needs to be reduced, or the nipple repositioned to a more natural male position.

## 3. THE SUTURES

Male breast reduction surgery incisions are closed with dissolvable sutures, so they will not need to be removed post-op. Sometimes, a tiny plastic tube is inserted to drain off any excess fluids. This will be removed a few days after the gynecomastia surgery. The closed incisions are normally then covered with a dressing and the chest may be wrapped to keep the skin firmly in place while it heals.

## 4. THE RESULTS

The results of male breast reduction surgery are immediately visible. Over time, post-surgical swelling will subside and resolve, and incision lines will gradually refine in appearance.

# Recovery and healing

Gynecomastia recovery times vary from patient to patient. You will feel some discomfort after surgery—this may last from a few days to several weeks and can be controlled by prescription medications from your doctor. It is also quite common to experience a little numbness from bruised nerves in and around your breast area. Most of this should pass over time, as you heal.

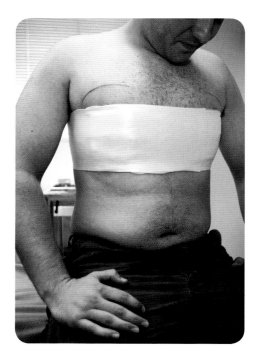

You should arrange to have someone drive you home after your surgery and to help you out for a day or two if needed. You will need to wear a compression garment continuously for 1–2 weeks, and at night for a few weeks after that. The worst of your swelling will go down in the first few weeks but it may be 3 months or more before the final results of your surgery become apparent.

You can return to work as soon as you feel well enough. This could be as early as a day or two after surgery. Your surgeon may advise you to avoid sex for 1–2 weeks, and heavy exercise for about 3 weeks. You will also be warned to avoid any sport or job that risks a blow to the chest area for at least 4 weeks. It will take about 1 month before you are able to resume all your normal activities after male breast reduction surgery.

Avoid exposing your scars to the sun for at least 6 months, as they may turn dark permanently in the sunshine. If you must expose this skin, wear a total sun block.

**After male breast reduction surgery a compression garment will be worn for up to several weeks.**

# FACTS
## MALE BREAST REDUCTION

| | |
|---|---|
| **Description** | Surgery to remove excess fat and/or glandular tissue and skin; may be suitable for men who feel self-conscious about their "man breasts". |
| **Length of surgery** | 2–3 hours |
| **In/outpatient** | Outpatient |
| **Anesthesia** | Local or general |
| **Back to work in...** | Within days |
| **Back to the gym in...** | 1 month |
| **Treatment frequency** | Once or more as desired |
| **Risks** | • Swelling, tenderness, numbness, and bruising<br>• Unfavorable scarring<br>• Hematoma<br>• Blood clots<br>• Infection<br>• Pigmentation changes<br>• Breast contour and shape irregularities<br>• Skin discoloration, permanent pigmentation changes, swelling, and bruising<br>• Damage to skin or internal organs<br>• Breast asymmetry<br>• Fat necrosis<br>• Fluid accumulation (seroma)<br>• Deep vein thrombosis, cardiac and pulmonary complications<br>• Pain, which may persist<br>• Possibility of revision surgery |
| **Duration of results** | Long-lasting |

# MALE TUMMY TUCK
*Abdominoplasty*

## WHY HAVE A TUMMY TUCK?

A common problem as men age is the development of "love handles," a "pot belly," or a "spare tire." Frequent or dramatic changes in weight can cause the abdominal muscles to weaken, the skin to sag, and stretch marks to appear. Male abdominoplasty is a common procedure that can reduce the size of a belly by removing excess skin and tightening the muscles in the midsection.

## *What is a male tummy tuck?*

For many men, this surgery can achieve a flatter, tighter, more aesthetically appealing abdominal contour. Men considering it should be aware that abdominoplasty is not a suitable treatment for obesity, nor should it be used in cases of small fat deposits where the skin retains its elasticity.

The ideal candidate for male abdominoplasty is a person who is close to their ideal body weight, but whose abdominal region does not respond well to diet and exercise. It is important for a male abdominoplasty patient to have a good understanding of what to expect before, during, and after the procedure.

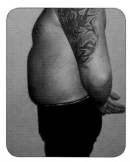

BEFORE

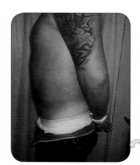

AFTER

Male tummy tuck surgery can create a flatter and tighter abdominal contour.

## FACTS
### MALE TUMMY TUCK

| | |
|---|---|
| **Description** | A procedure used to give a tighter, flatter stomach and reduce the appearance of stretch marks on the lower abdomen. |
| **Length of surgery** | 2–5 hours |
| **In/outpatient** | Inpatient |
| **Anesthesia** | General, or local plus sedation |
| **Back to work in...** | 2–4 weeks |
| **Back to the gym in...** | 6 weeks |
| **Treatment frequency** | Once or more as desired |
| **Risks** | • See page 157 |
| **Duration of results** | Long-lasting |

The surgery is performed by making an incision in the lower abdomen from hip to hip and a second incision to reposition the belly button. The abdominal muscles are tightened, excess skin and fat is removed, and the skin is stretched to create a firmer, smoother appearance. Sometimes a surgeon will employ liposuction techniques to remove excess fat from the area.

### MINI-ABDOMINOPLASTY

A mini-abdominoplasty consists of the same steps, however; a much smaller incision is made in the lower stomach region, the skin and fat of the lower abdomen are enhanced, but the navel is not repositioned.

For more information on tummy tuck surgery see pages 152–157.

# MALE FACELIFT
## *Rhytidectomy*

### FACELIFT SURGERY DEFINITION

Facelift procedures designed for men can be an effective way to minimize the unwanted effects of age, stress, and exposure to the sun. These include sagging in the cheeks and around the neck and jawline, which contributes to a heavy, congested look that most men find undesirable.

## *What is a male facelift?*

**Although the results achieved with male facelift surgery are similar to those enjoyed by women, there are differences in approach that potential patients should be aware of. Generally, men who are healthy but would like to enhance their appearance make good candidates for a male facelift. However, it is important to have a realistic notion of what to expect.**

A facelift for men involves the removal of facial fat and excess skin, along with the careful remodeling of distorted muscles and tissue below the facial surface. Certain specific techniques are used to optimize the aesthetic outcome for male patients.

Perhaps the key difference between facelift surgery for men and women concerns the incisions made during surgery. Because men tend to wear their hair shorter than women, hiding scars can be more difficult. This often allows for less flexibility in terms of where incisions can be made. However, they are always placed as inconspicuously as possible, often along the natural crease where the ear meets the side of the face, around the earlobe, and into the lower scalp area under the hair.

For more information on facelift surgery see pages 44–49.

**Shown here is a male "mini" facelift, also known as an "S lift-short scar" facelift.**

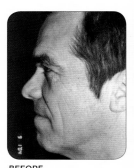
BEFORE

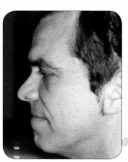
AFTER

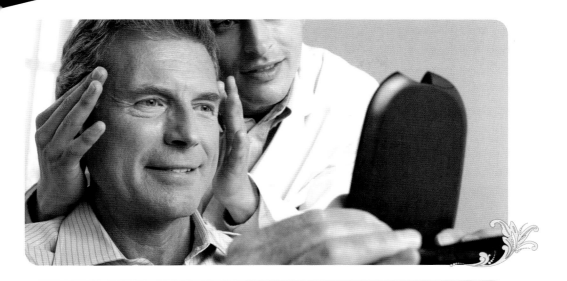

## FACTS
### MALE FACELIFT

| | |
|---|---|
| **Description** | The skin of the face is stretched back and up to give a fresher, more youthful appearance. |
| **Length of surgery** | 2–3 hours |
| **In/outpatient** | Inpatient |
| **Anesthesia** | General |
| **Back to work in...** | 4 weeks |
| **Back to the gym in...** | 6 weeks |
| **Treatment frequency** | Once or more as desired |
| **Risks** | • See page 49. |
| **Duration of results** | 5–10 years |

# MALE NOSE SURGERY
*Rhinoplasty*

## *What is male rhinoplasty?*

**Rhinoplasty for men is designed to change the shape and contour of the nose for both aesthetic and health-related reasons. While this surgery is primarily thought of as an aesthetic procedure, it can greatly help patients who have trouble breathing due to bone and cartilage defects and deformities. Male rhinoplasty candidates should be at least 16 years old, which is about the age when the nose stops growing.**

### WHY HAVE RHINOPLASTY?

Male rhinoplasty has become very popular. Rhinoplasty can alter the shape and contour of the nose; a source of embarrassment and self-consciousness for many men.

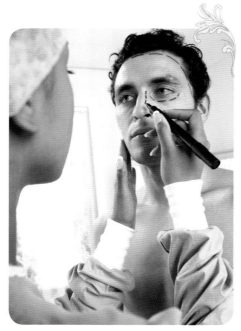

A good candidate may feel that his nose is either too large or too small in comparison to the rest of his face. He may also be unhappy with the appearance of the nasal tip if it droops, is bulbous, or protrudes.

By changing the contour and shape of different parts of the nose—the tip, the nostrils, or the bridge—as well as by adjusting the overall size, symmetry, and orientation of the nose, rhinoplasty can provide men with very satisfying results. For some patients, the surgeon will recommend combining rhinoplasty with other cosmetic procedures such as a facelift or chin implants in order to bring about a much more dramatic and well-balanced facial change.

For more information on rhinoplasty, see pages 90–95.

# FACTS
## MALE NOSE SURGERY

| | |
|---|---|
| **Description** | Cosmetic procedure performed to enhance the appearance of the nose. |
| **Length of surgery** | 1–2 hours |
| **In/outpatient** | Outpatient |
| **Anesthesia** | General |
| **Back to work in...** | 7–10 days |
| **Back to the gym in...** | 2 weeks |
| **Treatment frequency** | Once |
| **Risks** | • See page 95 |
| **Duration of results** | Permanent |

# MALE LIPOSUCTION
*Lipoplasty*

## WHY HAVE LIPOSUCTION?

Liposuction can address a number of areas of the male body; it can be very helpful in reducing the appearance of "love handles," or excess fat around the abdominal area. Many men have a hard time losing weight in this area.

## What is male liposuction?

**Male liposuction is just the same as the procedure carried out on women. As a growing number of men turn to cosmetic surgery to improve their appearance, male liposuction promises to become an even more popular cosmetic surgery option.**

A common area of the body for male liposuction is the abdomen. Liposuction can also be an effective treatment for gynecomastia, or the abnormal enlargement of the male breast. While liposuction can often be used as a form of breast reduction in men, it is important that the surgeon first determines whether the excess tissue in the breast is fatty or glandular.

Liposuction for men is not just limited to the body: more and more, men are turning to liposuction to slim, sculpt, and rejuvenate their faces. Some common areas for male facial liposuction are the chin, neck, and jowls. Removing fat from these areas can restore definition to facial features and give the face an overall more youthful and refreshed appearance.

For more information on liposuction, see pages 132 to 151.

**Male liposuction can remove excess fat from the abdominal area.**

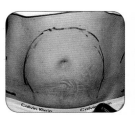
BEFORE

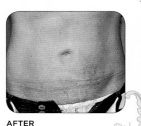
AFTER

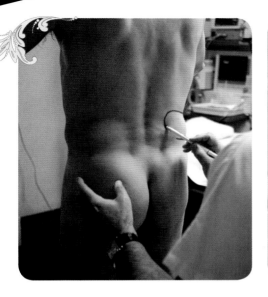
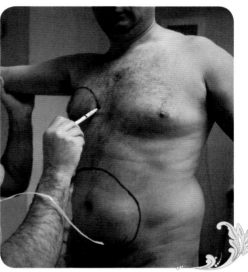

# FACTS
## MALE LIPOSUCTION

| | |
|---|---|
| **Description** | Fat is removed from specific areas of the body. |
| **Length of surgery** | Varies: from 1–2 hours per area treated |
| **In/outpatient** | Inpatient or outpatient |
| **Anesthesia** | General or twilight |
| **Back to work in...** | Varies |
| **Back to the gym in...** | Varies |
| **Treatment frequency** | Once or more as desired |
| **Risks** | • See page 139 |
| **Duration of results** | Long-lasting |

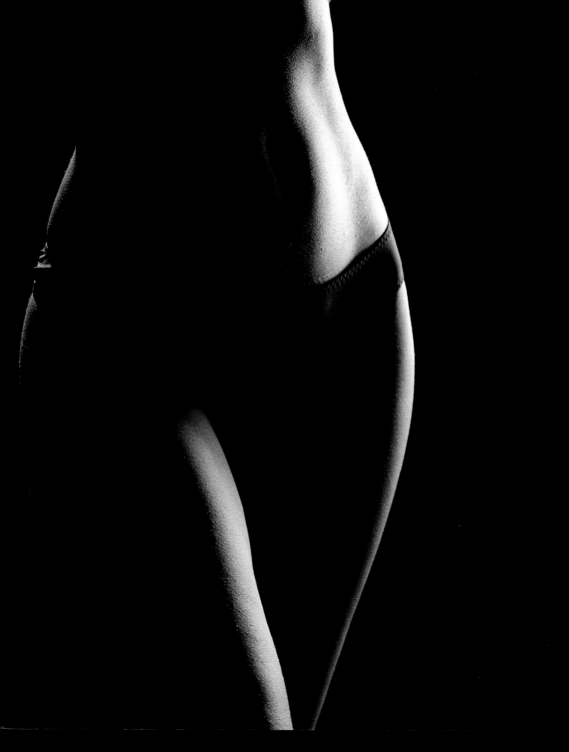

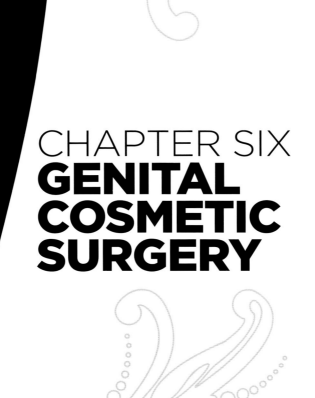

# CHAPTER SIX
# GENITAL COSMETIC SURGERY

# GENITAL COSMETIC SURGERY
*An overview*

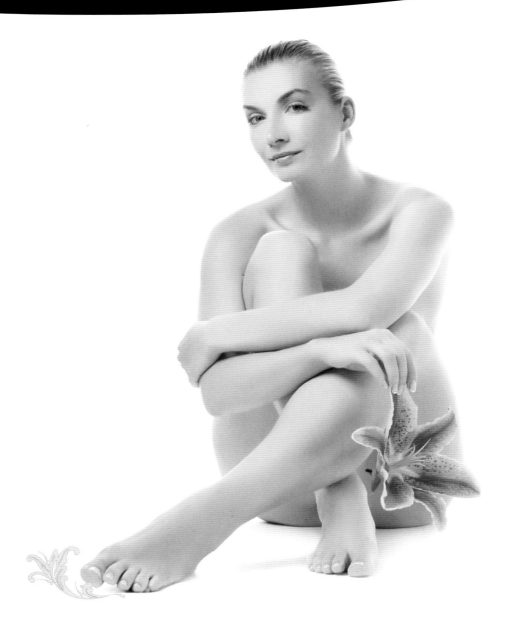

Many people are afraid to talk about so-called "embarrassing areas"; consequently, one of the least talked-about areas of cosmetic surgery is that of genital cosmetic surgery. All women are born with differently shaped genitalia, and with the effects of childbirth and age factored in, many suffer from problems and defects with their genitalia that can make them feel very self-conscious and unhappy, and can even affect relationships. However, there is surgery available to remedy these problems. For men unhappy with the size or shape of their penis, there are options to increase either the length of the penis, the girth, or both.

Female genital problems include oversized, elongated, or asymmetrical (lopsided) labia minora, the inner vaginal lips which surround the entrance to the vagina. This can cause irritation and discomfort when wearing particular clothes, doing certain activities (such as cycling and horse riding), or during sexual intercourse. Loose or weak vaginal muscles, mainly caused by childbirth, can cause problems for both the woman herself and her sexual partner during intercourse; pelvic floor exercises cannot correct this. Many women are now seeking cosmetic vaginal surgery to restore self-esteem and rejuvenate their love lives. Vaginal reconstruction (not covered here) is in the form of vaginoplasty (vaginal rejuvenation and tightening) while labia surgery is in the form of labiaplasty (labia reduction and beautification, see overleaf). Hymenoplasty (reconstruction of the hymen) returns the ruptured hymen to a pre-sexual state, and is not covered here.

Male patients should consider all the options very carefully before embarking on any treatment to increase penis length or girth. It may be worth discussing concerns with your family doctor, prior to making any decision. Penis enhancement surgery is still somewhat experimental and should only be considered as a last resort, taking into account not only the benefits but the potential risks and complications too. Aside from medical reasons, doctors resort to penis surgery to meet the psychological or aesthetic needs of men. This need arises when either men themselves or their sexual partners are not satisfied with the size of the penis.

# LABIAPLASTY
*Labia rejuvenation*

## WHY HAVE LABIAPLASTY?

A labiaplasty may be performed to surgically reshape or reduce the external appearance of the vagina on women who are unhappy with the appearance of their labia.

## What is labiaplasty?

**Enlarged inner genital lips (labia minora) may hang down outside the vagina as a result of becoming loose or stretched. The excess skin may present hygiene problems or make sexual intercourse and other activities such as cycling, walking, or sitting uncomfortable. The patient may also be embarrassed about the appearance of their labia, and their self-confidence may suffer as a result.**

## Am I a candidate for labiaplasty?

The procedure is suitable for any woman over 18 who is physically and emotionally healthy and wants to be more comfortable with the shape and feeling of her genitalia.

**Suitable candidates for labia rejuvenation surgery include women who:**
- Experience problems with sexual intercourse or have labia pain
- Are uncomfortable when sitting, cycling, or walking due to enlarged labia
- Would like to improve the appearance of their labia
- Have been born with large, asymmetrical, or protruding labia

- Experience emotional discomfort and self-esteem issues due to the appearance of their labia
- Are not planning to have any more children
- Have realistic expectations for the outcome of their labiaplasty.

**Unsuitable candidates for labiaplasty include women who:**
- Are pregnant or menstruating
- Have episiotomy complications
- Have a yeast infection or herpes virus
- Have bladder incontinence
- Have a prolapsed uterus.

## The basic procedure

During the labiaplasty, the surgeon removes the excess tissue of the labia minora, and the labia majora (on the outside of the body) may also be reduced by surgery or liposuction.

### 1. ANESTHESIA
Local, twilight, or general anesthesia will be administered. Your doctor will determine the best choice for you.

### 2. THE INCISION AND RESHAPING
One of two techniques may be used next: a long strip of the labia minora is excised (cut away), or alternatively, a wedge-shaped section is cut away which removes a V-shaped area of the labia minora. The excess is removed and the top and bottom are brought together. Excess skin or fat from the labia majora is removed with liposuction.

### 3. THE SUTURES
Dissolvable sutures are used to close the incision.

### 4. THE RESULTS
The results of your labiaplasty procedure will be immediately obvious. The results are permanent, though it is possible for the labia to become stretched again through pregnancy and childbirth or sexual activity.

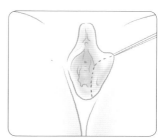

POSITION OF INCISION

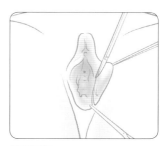

INCISION

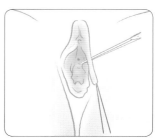

RESHAPING

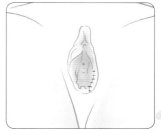

SUTURING

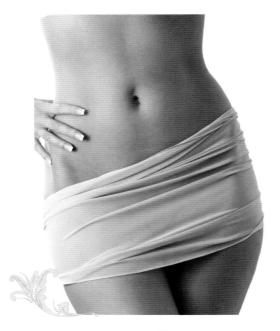

## Preparing for labiaplasty

You can prepare for your labiaplasty procedure by keeping to a healthy diet and lifestyle, to aid strength and recovery. During your consultation you should inform your cosmetic surgeon if you smoke or take medication and you will be advised accordingly.

## Recovery and healing

Mild to moderate discomfort and swelling will often be experienced by women after undergoing labiaplasty. Take presribed pain medication. Discomfort should subside within several days but mild discomfort can continue for several weeks. You may need to wear supportive undergarments to help reduce swelling, which should subside within 6 weeks. Depending on the type of sutures used and their location, they should dissolve within 7 to 21 days.

You may be advised to avoid intercourse for 3–6 weeks following labiaplasty, and may also be told to avoid using tampons and vaginal douches during your recovery period. Labiaplasty patients should be able to return to work and normal activities within 2–5 days, and more strenuous activities within 2–3 weeks.

# FACTS
## LABIAPLASTY SURGERY

| | |
|---|---|
| **Description** | Surgery to reshape or reduce the external appearance of the vagina. |
| **Length of surgery** | 1 hour |
| **In/outpatient** | Outpatient |
| **Anesthesia** | General or twilight |
| **Back to work in...** | 2–5 days |
| **Back to the gym in...** | 2–3 weeks |
| **Treatment frequency** | Once |
| **Risks** | • Scarring<br>• Infection<br>• Asymmetry of the labia<br>• Pigmentation changes<br>• Changes in sensation<br>• Changes in texture or pigment of the labial edge<br>• Separation of the labial edge |
| **Duration of results** | Long-lasting |

# PENIS ENLARGEMENT
## Penis widening / lengthening

## What is penis enlargement?

According to the American Urological Association, the techniques and procedures used in penis enlargement surgery have not yet been proven through research studies to be entirely effective or safe. It is not known whether the potential benefits of the penile surgery outweigh the possible dangers associated with it. This is something the patient considering the surgery must decide after careful consideration and extensive consultation with a board-certified surgeon experienced in penis enlargement surgery.

## Penis enlargement: the options

Before making the decision to have penis enlargement surgery, whether it be penis widening or penis lengthening (or both), it is essential that you discuss all of the complications that could arise after the surgery with a cosmetic surgeon. You should make the surgeon aware of your medical history as well as any allergies that you have. It is important that you have realistic objectives about the outcome of penis enlargement surgery, as this will contribute to the overall result and success of your treatment. There are a number of options available:

### INFLATABLE IMPLANTS

The corpora cavernosa (a pair of sponge-like regions of erectile tissue which contain most of the blood in the penis during erection) are replaced with inflatable penile implants. This is performed primarily as a therapeutic surgery for men suffering from complete impotence; this surgery consists of an implanted pump placed in the groin, which can be manipulated by hand to fill these cylinders from an implanted reservoir in order to achieve an erection. The replacement cylinders are normally sized to be direct replacements for the corpus cavernosa, but larger ones can be implanted. However, the result is an uncomfortable stretching of the other penile tissues, which can have a number of complications.

## LIGAMENT CUTTING

Another surgical option is to cut the basal penile ligament, which can result in an apparent lengthening of the penis by up to 2 inches (5 cm) in some patients. With this procedure, while the penis elongates and hardens with an erection, it can no longer become truly erect, but only hangs. The results of this surgery vary greatly between individuals, with some men reporting no measurable lengthening at all.

## PENILE INJECTION

This cosmetic surgery procedure takes fat cells from elsewhere in the body and injects them below the surface of the skin of the shaft of the penis to increase its thickness (but not length). The penile shaft normally has little or no fat, and this method results in an unnatural appearance and feel, as well as risking radical shifting of the fat injected. Another method involves injection of liquid silicone into the penis and scrotum. This technique can cause enormous increases in the girth of the penis (increasing the penis volume by over 900 percent) but is irreversible. Side effects including loss of sensation, inability to carry out penetrative intercourse, scarring, and deformation.

## Risks and complications

As with all surgical procedures there are potential risks.

- Some patients will report a decrease in the size of their penis when it is in the erect and upward position.
- Some patients will notice a keloid scar developing at the surgical site (keloids are firm, rubbery lesions or shiny, fibrous nodules, and can vary from pink to flesh-colored or red to dark brown in color).
- There are rare instances where the incisions on the skin separate thus

- causing an infection to develop.
- Some patients experience a certain amount of bleeding and bruising as well as swelling of their penis but these are all temporary conditions.
- In some cases the patient will find that their penis is lacking in sensation and experience erectile dysfunction; this is sometimes a temporary effect of penile lengthening surgery.
- Another rare side effect is when serum accumulates under the skin.

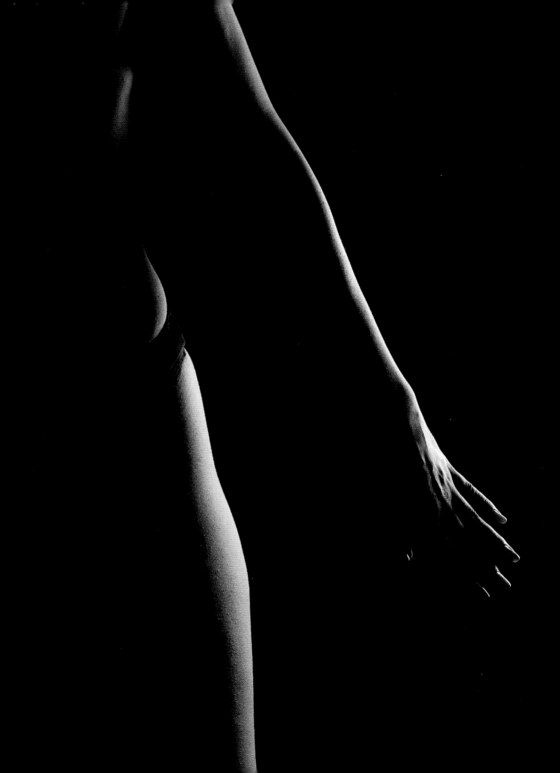

# CHAPTER SEVEN
## NONSURGICAL PROCEDURES

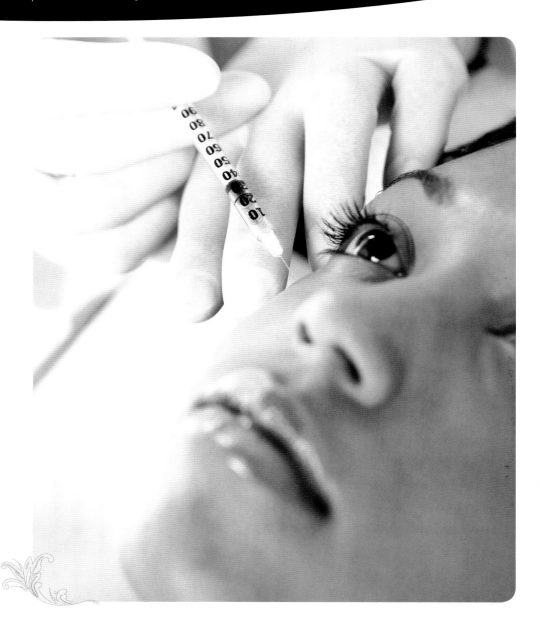

**Non-invasive or minimally invasive procedures are cosmetic beauty treatments for individuals who want to improve the appearance of an aspect of their face and/or body, but do not wish to undergo the risk of complications, side effects, and long recovery times associated with more invasive cosmetic surgery procedures.**

The distinguishing difference between non-invasive cosmetic surgery and other forms of cosmetic surgery is that it isn't really surgery at all. While a tummy tuck requires anesthesia and "going under the knife," a Botox treatment requires only an injection.

For those who are not confident enough to undergo a surgical procedure, but who want to make aesthetic improvements, there are many benefits in choosing non-invasive over invasive cosmetic surgery. Some procedures can be done within a few hours, with minimal swelling and redness. Scars are also very uncommon and you would not need to take a lot of time off from work to heal. Anesthesia and overnight hospital stays are not a requirement, which means the price of non-invasive procedures is much lower than for invasive surgery.

## POPULAR TREATMENTS

Popular treatments include laser hair removal and skin rejuvenation techniques. Non-invasive procedures can treat problematic areas of the face and body including sagging skin, cellulite, localized deposits of fat, skin wrinkles, irregularities, and blemishes, and excess hair. Chemical peels can also be applied to the face and neck, giving the skin a tighter, younger appearance.

Many people in their late twenties onward are opting for nonsurgical treatments, as they fit well within a busy schedule, are affordable, and produce results that can last up to several months.

Each individual procedure varies in time and technique. Different techniques include injectable fillers and toxins, lasers, lights, and radio frequency (RF) technology.

So, how do you know which one to choose? It is essential that you consult either a qualified surgeon or dermatologist before consenting to undergo any cosmetic procedure. They will be able to give you detailed advice regarding your specific skin texture, tone, and elasticity. As certain treatments are not recommended for all skin types, you will know exactly what to avoid by talking directly to the experts. They will also be able to recommend the number of treatments that will be suitable for you. Some procedures require only one visit to the clinic before significant results are visible; however more often than not, a course of several treatments is required, depending on the severity of the skin problem and the type of skin being treated.

## CHOOSING A PRACTITIONER

It is a good idea to ask friends and family if they would recommend a particular surgeon or clinic, as first-hand experience from someone you know and trust can be extremely helpful.

Price and quality of aftercare are also very important when it comes to choosing both your type of treatment and the person performing it. Enquire at a few different clinics and try to get the best possible deal.

Make sure you ask how experienced your practitioner is, and how often they perform the procedure. It is also advisable to see plenty of before and after pictures, so that you have a realistic idea of what to expect post treatment. Most good surgeons or clinical staff will do their best to put you at ease, and will give you a detailed idea of what to expect before the actual procedure occurs. If however, you feel uncomfortable or start having second thoughts, it may be worthwhile visiting another clinic to see where you would prefer to receive treatment. The layout and ambience of a clinic can hugely impact your comfort level, and the friendliness of staff can either give you peace of mind or make you even more anxious. Because the human body doesn't heal well under stress, it is advisable to go for the clinic where you feel happiest, and the surgeon you trust most with your face or body.

You should receive plenty of information regarding which painkillers to use, and which sort of aftercare regime to follow. Some procedures leave your skin feeling raw and sensitive, so extra care and specialist products may be needed to keep it clean and healthy. It is also highly recommended that you conduct a patch test before proceeding with the full treatment, as there is no way of knowing how your skin will react.

## BEFORE THE PROCEDURE

Surgery of any kind is a big decision, so make sure you are clear about the side effects and possible complications that may be involved. Nonsurgical cosmetic procedure side effects and risks vary from patient to patient. Though generally mild, they can include redness, swelling, blisters, bumps, and rare cases of surface irregularities.

It may also be advisable to opt for a combination of invasive and non-invasive procedures. While surgery can remove excess skin from the face and body, nonsurgical cosmetic treatments can leave it looking fresh, young, and positively edible. Although their results don't last as long as those from invasive surgery, non-invasive treatments are more affordable, less painful, and are becoming increasingly popular. If you wish to be "bikini-beautiful" all year round, but don't want to spend a fortune on full body contouring, then non-invasive treatments can be a great alternative.

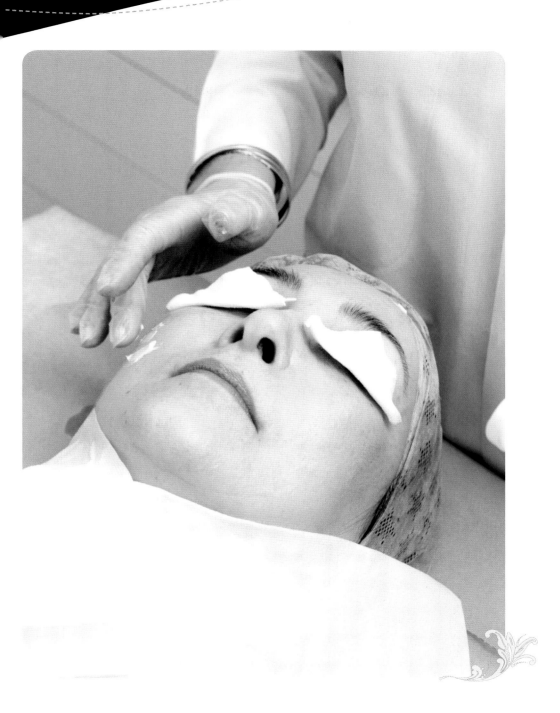

# FILLERS AND TOXINS
*Botox and injectables*

## BOTOX OR FILLER?

Every time a new injectable arrives on the market it gets labeled the "new Botox." However it is important to understand that Botox is not a filler. Botox relaxes muscles to make lines disappear and can help in the prevention of new lines forming. Fillers, on the other hand, temporarily plump up creases and lines but cannot prevent new lines or creases forming.

## Which treatment?

**Fillers allow your muscles to remain fully active, whereas Botox does not. Fillers are ideal for adding volume to the face, which Botox cannot do, and fillers work best in deep creases, cheeks, and in the lips. These two treatments often work well in tandem and are not mutually exclusive.**

## BOTOX

Botox (the tradename of botulinum toxin type A) is the fastest growing cosmetic procedure in the United States. Botox cosmetic injection is a simple procedure in which the surgeon carefully injects a low dose of the toxin into an individual's facial muscles, causing temporary relaxation of the injected area.

Doctors first used botulinum toxin as a relaxant to treat muscle disorders, before realizing its cosmetic potential. Pioneered for cosmetic use in 1987, botulinum toxin is a purified form of one of the world's most poisonous substances. However, when carefully injected by cosmetic surgeons in minute doses, botulinum toxin type A can reduce the signs of aging. Botox was

approved for cosmetic use by the Food and Drug Administration (FDA) in 2002.

Cosmetic uses for Botox include treating common signs of aging such as horizontal lines on the forehead, vertical lines between the eyebrows and on the bridge of the nose, and fine lines and "crow's feet" at the corners of the eyes. Botox injections are non-invasive and require little or no recovery time.

Botox typically reduces wrinkles by 80 percent. Patients are usually between the ages of 35 and 60, and results will vary from person to person. The treatment takes just a few minutes, and during the procedure very small doses of Botox are injected into the muscles underneath the wrinkled area to be treated. The exact location of the injection

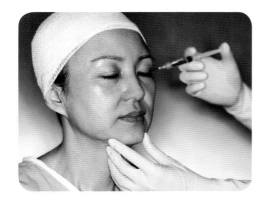

depends on the location, size, and typical use of the muscles. The Botox procedure does not usually require anesthesia, although sometimes an anesthetic cream will be applied to the area to be treated.

The Botox then binds to the nerve ending, which in turn virtually blocks the release of the chemical acetylcholine that is released by the nerve cells. This blocks electrical signals for the muscles to contract and move. The injected muscle is paralyzed or weakened, then it relaxes, creating a smooth surface and reducing the appearance of the wrinkles and lines on the skin, though the surrounding muscles remain unaffected.

This smoothing effect lasts around 3–4 months, before the muscle recovers its original strength. However, due to the way Botox works, even when the effects have worn off, the remaining lines will not be as deep as before.

Botox procedures last about half an hour, and the results are most noticeable 1–2 weeks after the procedure. Botox results last around 3–6 months. The effects can be maintained by "top-up" injections two or three times a year.

While Botox treatments don't completely eradicate the signs of aging, they can significantly reduce the appearance of moderate to severe frown lines, smooth wrinkles, and prevent new wrinkles from forming. Skin often appears smoother and more youthful after Botox injections.

Botox can be a beneficial cosmetic "middle ground" for patients who do not want to undergo invasive cosmetic surgery such as facelift yet who need treatment that is more effective than creams. For people in their twenties, thirties, and older, Botox treatment can postpone or eliminate the need for more invasive facial cosmetic procedures in the future such as surgery or laser resurfacing.

There are many practitioners who perform Botox injections, and it is very important that you consult a qualified, experienced doctor with extensive experience in administering Botox injections, to avoid risks and complications during and after your treatment.

## Where to start

If you are having Botox for the first time, start with small areas such as the frozen lines (gabella) or the crow's feet around the eyes, or the lines across your forehead which are horizontal, a little at a time will ensure you build up confidence with this treatment.

## INJECTABLE FILLERS

Injectable fillers are a practical way to address the early signs of aging, but not all injectable fillers are created equal... Fillers fall into two main categories: absorbable (temporary) and non-absorbable (permanent). The former are gradually broken down by the body, while the latter are not. Temporary fillers include hyaluronic acid and collagens, poly-L-lactic acid, and fat.

Permanent fillers carry more controversy with them, as injectable liquid silicone and semipermanent fillers including hybrid fillers also fall into this category. The general directive is that the longer filler is deemed to last, the greater the risk associated with it.

Temporary absorbable fillers that dissolve over time are generally considered to be the safest substances to opt for. A reputable cosmetic surgeon or dermatologist will be able to advise you which filler would best suit your individual needs.

Injectable fillers can cause side effects such as hardening, lumps and small bumps, bruises, swelling and redness, inflammation, rashes, migration, extrusion, allergic reaction, acne, and infection; although these do not occur with every person it is advisable to do your research on the product suggested to you by your doctor so that you are aware of the side effects and risks.

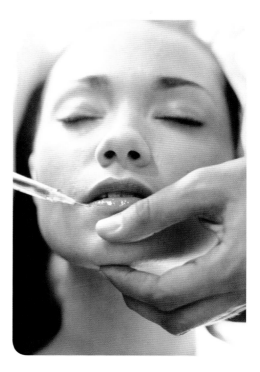

## INJECTABLE FILLER WITHOUT THE PAIN!

The future trend for injectable fillers is set to include pain relief in the syringe! Juvederm Ultra™ and Elevess™ are the first hyaluronic acid gel fillers with pain relief in the syringe. Puragen® Plus and other brandnames such as Restylane are also set to follow the trend.

# Temporary filler options

## HYALURONIC ACID FILLERS

Hyaluronic acid is a natural substance found in all living organisms. High concentrations are found in soft connective tissue and in the fluid surrounding the eye. In skin tissue, hyaluronic acid is a jello-like substance that fills the space between collagen and elastin fibers. It is also present in some cartilage and joint fluids.

Hyaluronic acid hydrates the skin by holding in water; aids the transport of essential nutrients from the bloodstream to living skin cells; and acts as a cushioning and lubricating agent against mechanical and chemical damage. Due to the natural aging process and other factors including pollutants, sunlight, fatigue, and hormonal changes, the body's natural store of hyaluronic acid is degraded and destroyed over time, leading to facial furrows and wrinkles.

Dermal fillers are made of various kinds of natural and manmade or synthetic materials. Over the last 30 years, synthetic forms of hyaluronic acid have been developed and used to correct medical disorders, but now synthetic forms of hyaluronic acid are being manufactured in injectable gel form for use in facial enhancement.

**Brand names for hyaluronic acid fillers currently include:** Restylane® • Juvederm Ultra™ • Elevess™ • Prevelle® • Teosysal® • Belotero®

## COLLAGEN FILLERS

Collagen is a natural, essential protein complex that occurs in the human body, is found in skin, muscle, tendons, and bones and provides structural support. Collagen molecules form fibrils that produce necessary fibers for our bodies. The configuration of fibers is the foundation for tissue formation and forms a fibrous network on which new cells can grow. Through the natural processes of aging, collagen in the dermis is gradually lost, and it is this that contributes to the formation of facial lines.

Collagen fillers are classified as follows:

- Collagen fillers that use human collagen much like that found in skin. Human collagen implants are highly purified and isolated from human skin grown in a laboratory.
- Collagen fillers that are bovine-based or mammal-based. Injectable bovine collagen is made of sterile, purified collagen from cow skin.

**Brand names for collagen fillers currently include:** Evolence™
- Zyderm ® • Zyplast®
- Cosmoderm® • Cosmoplast®

## POLYMER FILLERS

Polymer fillers are a new category of fillers emerging in the footsteps of the hyaluronic acids and collagens that preceded them.

# Semi-permanent filler options

## SCULPTRA®

A unique product that is considered to be more of a "volumizing" injectable, rather than a wrinkle filler, Sculptra is considered a good substitute for fat injections. It is made of poly-L-lactic acid, a material that has been used previously over a long period of time in dissolvable stitches. When injected it adds volume to depressed areas such as hollow areas around eye sockets, temples, and the mouth area, and it is especially effective for concave cheeks. It has also been used on the décolleté area. It works by increasing the thickness of the skin and by stimulating the body to produce new collagen. A series of at least three treatments is needed for full correction and effectiveness; this also depends on the areas requiring treatment.

## RADIESSE®

Radiesse is a product made up of calcium hydroxylapatite which is made up of calcium and phosphate. It is the same mineral component found in bones and teeth, so is very biocompatible. In time the tiny microspheres break down and are absorbed into the body. Radiesse is injected deep into the dermis and can smooth out nose-to-mouth lines (nasolabial folds), marionette lines, depressed scars, and the chin area; it can also be effective for cheek enhancement, to fill in scars, and to treat some nasal defects.

## FAT INJECTIONS

Fat injections, in simple terms, can be considered the "recycling of fat" which is a particularly interesting concept as it does actually work... Fat is extracted by syringe from the hips, tummy, or thighs—or wherever else available—and is then cleansed and re-injected into facial folds, creases, lips, or hollows. The two-step procedure of first harvesting the fat from the patient then re-injecting can be performed along with facial surgery or as a standalone procedure. Swelling and redness can last for several days and bruising is likely as there is more trauma and manipulation required by the cosmetic surgeon or doctor than is normally required with commercially available fillers.

# Permanent filler options

Permanent fillers are considered to be more "risky" than their short-term alternatives. Permanent fillers will remain in your body and the results cannot be reversed. They will not be naturally absorbed into the body.

## ARTEFILL®

ArteFill is a gel dermal filler consisting of millions of synthetic microspheres (Polymethyl-methacrylate or PMMA) suspended in purified bovine (derived from cows) collagen. ArteFill also contains the local anesthetic lidocaine to reduce discomfort during injection. Men and women of any age may receive ArteFill treatment. Ideal candidates may have already tried temporary injections, are sure of the results that they want to achieve, and are sure they want a permanent result. ArteFill is not suitable for people with allergies to bovine collagen or patients with chronic skin infections. ArteFill is not recommended for areas of thinner skin, such as laughter lines around the eyes. It is used for acne scars, nasolabial folds, lips, and the building up of the cheek area, as well as chin contours.

## BIO-ALCAMID®

Bio-Alcamid is an injectable facial implant. The main ingredient is a gel comprising 96 percent water and 4 percent synthetic reticulate polymer called a polyacrylamide. After being injected into the skin a capsule is formed that encloses the substance so that it forms an implant; it is then massaged and manipulated into the place where it's needed.

## BIOINBLUE®

This is a synthetic hydrogel consisting of 6 percent polyvinyl and alcohol (called PVA) and 94 percent non-pirogenic water. It has a soft consistency because of its high water content and is often used within the lips.

## INJECTABLE LIQUID SILICONE

Silicone has been used as a permanent filler since the 1940s; however it has been misused over time and as a consequence its use is controversial. For a long time it was no longer used, however, liquid silicone droplets seems to be making a comeback. Silicone is permanent and this means once it is in, it will last forever, which has its pros and cons. For more information on injectable silicone, ask a cosmetic surgeon or a dermatologist to explain the process and the possible risks, complications, and side effects.

# SKIN RESURFACING
## *Chemical peel / microdermabrasion / lasers*

### SKIN RESURFACING DEFINITION

"Skin resurfacing" is a term that covers a range of treatments, from chemical peels (where acid is applied to the skin) to microdermabrasion (mechanically rubbing away dead skin cells) and laser treatments.

## *What can they achieve?*

**Skin resurfacing treatments are designed to improve the appearance of the skin in a number of ways. They can remove old, dead skin cells and promote new cell growth. They can help to reduce the appearance of sun damage, age spots, fine lines and wrinkles, and other blemishes. Many leave the face with a "healthy glow."**

## *Skin resurfacing: the options*

### CHEMICAL PEEL

During a chemical peel, an acid solution is "painted" onto the skin to remove the outer layer of cells, lightly exfoliating the skin to give a healthy glow. There are three types of chemical face peel available— superficial chemical peel, medium-depth chemical peel, and deep chemical peel. Chemical facial peels can't alter the size of pores, improve sagging skin, or remove deep scarring, but the treatment can reduce fine wrinkles, freckles, and irregular pigmentation and remove sunspots and rough, scaly patches on the patient's skin.

Chemical peels are designed to accelerate the removal of old, dead skin cells at the surface of the skin to promote new cell growth, and can be used to treat a particular area (such as lines around the eyes or mouth), or all over the face, arms, hands, and neck. Chemical peels are normally safest and most effective when performed on the face.

Chemical facial peels can take anything from a few minutes to 2 hours, depending on the type of peel that you are having. Usually a series of four to six very superficial chemical peels are needed to treat aging skin and acne scars. For deep scars and lines and wrinkles one or two medium chemical face peels may be needed.

## MICRODERMABRASION

Microdermabrasion removes the uppermost layer of dead skin cells from the face, chest, and hands by mechanical abrasion. Microdermabrasion diminishes sun damage, fine lines and wrinkles, enlarged pores, blemishes, whiteheads and blackheads, and coarse-textured skin, for a more youthful appearance. Microdermabrasion treatment takes about 20–30 minutes and is sometimes called a "lunchtime peel" because there is little or no recovery time.

Microdermabrasion uses a powerful device to spray microcrystals of very fine, hard, sandlike aluminum dioxide across the skin's surface, which blasts away the uppermost layer of dead skin cells, exposing the skin beneath, promoting the growth of new, fresh skin and stimulating the production of collagen.

Microdermabrasion can be uncomfortable, but is not normally painful. Your doctor may recommend a series of four to six treatments for the best results, with healing time in between.

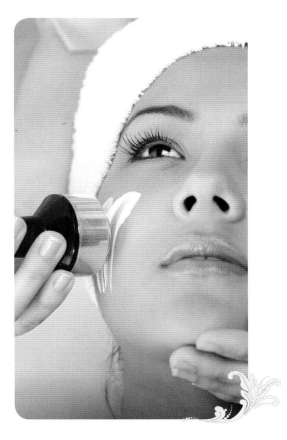

## LASERS

Laser skin resurfacing is a treatment to resurface your skin, or to improve the texture and overall appearance of your skin. It is a relatively new method of improving skin texture and appearance. Laser facial resurfacing can improve the appearance of fine lines and wrinkles of the entire face, or those that develop in specific regions of the face, such as the upper lip and around the eyes, as well as treating pigmentation disorders, such as sun and age spots.

Laser facial resurfacing can provide the doctor with more control over the penetration of the skin than other resurfacing treatments. Laser skin resurfacing allows doctors to treat delicate facial areas very precisely, such as those around your eyes and lips, as the laser gives the doctor more control over the penetration of the skin.

In addition to skin resurfacing, laser resurfacing is also used to remove facial scars, acne scars, and excess facial hair.

**Conditions that can be treated with laser facial resurfacing include:**

- Facial wrinkles, both static (wrinkles that do not change with facial movements) and dynamic (expression lines that may appear as folds when the skin is not moving, and deepen with facial muscular activity)
- Pigmentation resulting from sun exposure—freckles, sun spots, melasma (dark brown or gray irregular patches on the face), or other darkened patches of skin
- Scars—as the result of acne or injury to the skin
- Vascular conditions—small blood vessels visible on the surface of the skin, which may appear as facial thread veins or a red flush
- Loss of skin tone—weakening of collagen and elastin fibers.

A laser skin resurfacing procedure takes from just a few minutes to an hour and a half, depending on the size of the area being treated and the severity of the skin condition. During the laser resurfacing procedure, an intense beam of light energy is directed at the area to be treated. This laser beam destroys the outer layer of skin and at the same time heats the underlying skin, which stimulates the growth of new collagen fibers. As the wound heals, new skin forms, which is smoother and tighter.

## INTENSE PULSED LIGHT THERAPY (IPL)

IPL works by emitting a range of different wavelengths in each pulse of light. These target areas in the skin that are different in color to the surrounding tissue, such as scars, freckles, some birthmarks, and other areas of pigmented skin.

Your doctor will focus the intense pulsed light onto the area around the scar or blemish to be treated. IPL targets the lower levels of skin without affecting the upper levels, which means that any peeling and recovery time is normally reduced.

Treatment sessions usually last around 20 minutes, and you can usually return home immediately after treatment. A course of four to six treatments may be required to achieve the desired results.

If would like to reduce facial scars, blemishes, or certain skin conditions, IPL can provide an effective treatment. It can be used to treat acne scars and scarring due to injuries, or rosacea, port wine stains, sun damage, and age spots.

## LED PHOTOREJUVENATION

Light therapy or phototherapy consists of exposure to specific wavelengths of light using lasers, LEDs, fluorescent lamps, or very bright, full-spectrum lights, for a prescribed amount of time. LED photorejuvenation has proven effective in treating acne, seasonal affective disorder, and for some people it has ameliorated

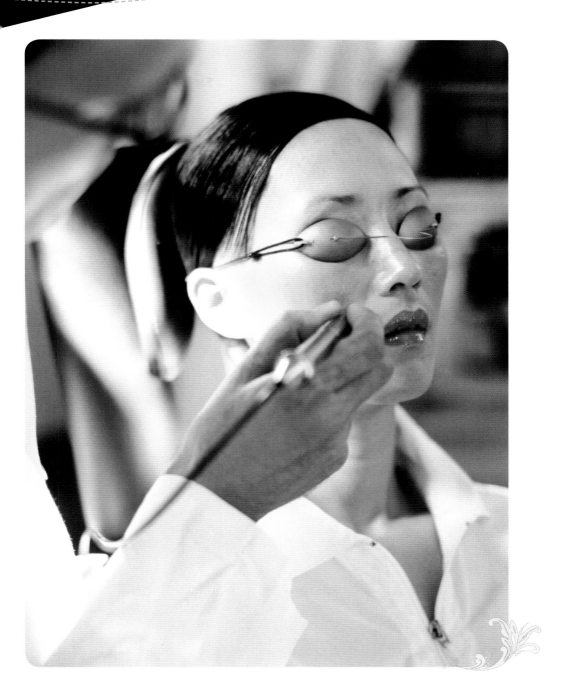

delayed sleep-phase syndrome. Light therapy or phototherapy also claims demonstrable benefits for skin conditions such as psoriasis.

Ion therapy stimulates the skin's fibroblasts to produce collagen and elastin proteins and is known for its deep cleansing properties, while light therapy is the most advanced non-invasive system available to diminish the appearance of fine lines, wrinkles, creases, furrows, and crow's feet.

## PHOTO PNEUMATIC THERAPY (PPx)

PPx uses a combination of pressure and broadband light to treat the skin. Unwanted red or brown pigment and unsightly veins are quickly and painlessly destroyed, leaving the skin with a fresh and youthful look. The treatment action removes melanin within the skin, which the body naturally and safely absorbs and destroys.

During a treatment with PPx you will feel a gentle and warm sensation as your skin

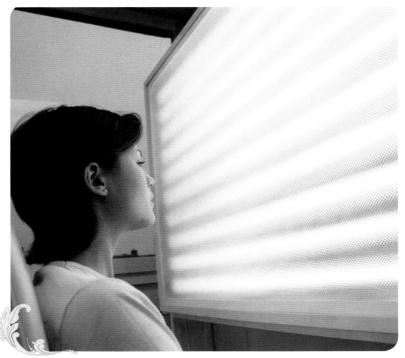

**LED photo-rejuvenation consists of exposure to specific wavelengths of light using lasers.**

is drawn into the treatment tip of the PPx device. A very gentle light energy will be applied to the treatment area, immediately after which you will feel your skin being gently released back into normal position. Patients describe the sensation as being similar to that of a warm massage. Facial rejuvenation usually takes 5 minutes, while treating a larger area such as arms for sun damage usually takes about 10 minutes.

## FRACTIONAL LASERS

Fractional lasers are resurfacing devices. There are now many systems that can produce fractional results; Fraxel® was the first to be introduced.

Fraxel uses laser technology applied to the skin to improve skin tone, smooth out fine lines, and even out skin discoloration by treating tiny sections of the skin, leaving the healthy surrounding skin undamaged and able to support the healing process.

A Fraxel procedure causes collagen (the protein that provides structure and support to the skin) to regenerate, while not affecting the undamaged parts of the skin's surface. The handheld Fraxel laser device delivers energy into the deeper layers of the skin in thousands of small dots (similar to pixels that make up the images on a screen), leaving the surrounding areas unaffected. These unaffected areas help speed up the healing process while the treated areas improve in appearance and underlying function.

Unlike conventional laser resurfacing procedures, which affect the whole surface of the skin, not just the area being treated, Fraxel only treats minute areas of damaged skin just deep enough to stimulate significant collagen regeneration. This results in minimal risk and downtime.

Fraxel laser treatment can be performed on any part of the body. Sun-damaged skin, fine lines and wrinkles, and uneven skin tone can all be successfully treated with Fraxel laser resurfacing.

## PLASMA SKIN REGENERATION:

Portrait® Plasma is a treatment of fine to deep wrinkles, superficial skin lesions, and pre-cancerous skin growths. It can reduce or eliminate brown spots and wrinkling caused by the sun and repair hyper-pigmentation. Instead of employing a light laser, light treatment, or injection, Portrait® Plasma works by delivering millisecond pulses of nitrogen plasma energy to the skin's surface via a special handpiece that stimulates and produces new collagen, the building blocks for skin regeneration.

The handpiece transfers plasma energy onto the skin without any direct contact. This heats up the tissue with no burning. A full-face treatment usually takes less than 45 minutes, whereas a regional treatment can be as short as 5–10 minutes. Shortly after, improvements in skin texture and elasticity and diminished wrinkles should result in a more youthful appearance.

Since there is no open skin or wound, the chances of infection are dramatically reduced. Other benefits include compatibility with many skin types, less pain, less redness, and faster healing time over other procedures. Portrait® Plasma skin regeneration can be used to treat an entire face or a specific area.

# SKIN TIGHTENING
*An overview*

## What is the procedure?

**Laser skin tightening is a non-invasive, nonsurgical procedure that uses an infrared laser to tighten skin by heating the collagen under the skin's surface.**

## WHY HAVE SKIN TIGHTENING?

Laser skin tightening works to rejuvenate the skin by heating the deeper layers of collagen under the skin, while simultaneously cooling the skin's outer layers, using a handheld laser device. This reduces the appearance of wrinkles and loose skin for a more youthful appearance.

## LASER SKIN TIGHTENING

The effect of laser skin tightening is noticeable immediately after the treatment, with additional tightening occurring over the following months as more new collagen is produced to support the facial tissues and create a younger, smoother facial appearance. Laser skin tightening patients may need two or three treatments approximately 30 days apart to achieve optimum results. The procedure takes around 30 minutes to 1 hour.

Laser skin tightening is a viable alternative for people who are not ready for or who do not need invasive cosmetic surgery. Laser skin tightening has none of the expense, risk, and downtime associated with surgical cosmetic facial procedures.

Laser skin tightening treatment is a virtually pain-free procedure that can tighten and smooth the skin on any area of the face or body that may have lax or sagging skin, including the forehead, crow's feet, double chin, the neck, the abdomen, and the knees. The laser skin tightening procedure stimulates long-term collagen growth because the infrared technology is able to penetrate deeply under the dermis, allowing a greater degree of skin tightening.

**Skin tightening brandnames include:**
Thermage® • Titan® • Refirme™ • Aluma™

**Opposite: Laser skin tightening produces immediate effects as well as additional effects that occur over time.**

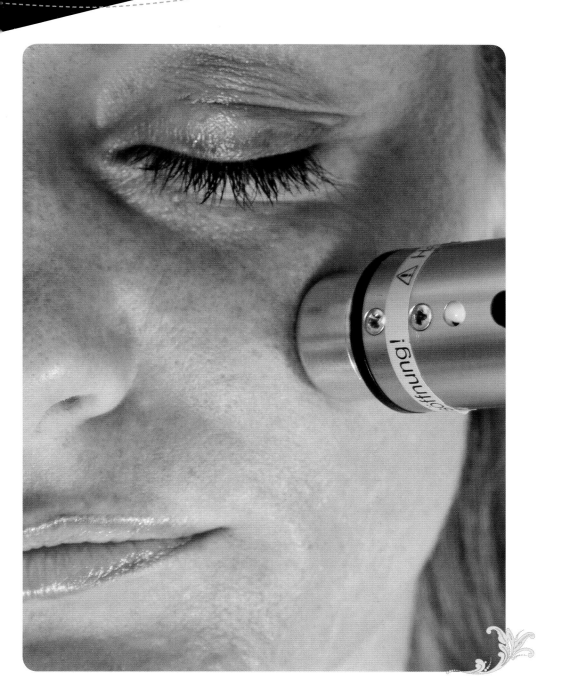

# CELLULITE TREATMENTS
*Velashape / Velasmooth / Endermologie / TriActive*

## WHAT IS CELLULITE?

Cellulite is a common problem for many women, whatever weight they may be. Cellulite has a dimpled, "cottage cheese" appearance, and is caused by an accumulation of fat and toxins that are trapped just beneath the surface of the skin.

## What is the procedure?

**Non-invasive treatments for cellulite make use of a combination of radio-frequency energy, infrared light, vacuum suction, mechanical massage, heating, cooling, and laser stimulation. The aim is to shrink and tighten the fat cells, tauten the skin, and encourage the drainage of fluid away from the problem areas.**

## Cellulite treatment: the options

### VELASHAPE®

Velashape is a procedure that uses radio frequency (RF) energy and infrared light to heat localized fatty tissue, while a vacuum and mechanical massage manipulates, smoothes, and tautens the skin.

Velashape reduces unsightly cellulite and the circumference of thighs, buttocks, arms, love handles, and the abdomen. The combination of infrared and RF energies is delivered through a handheld device that passes over the skin using rollers and a vacuum action. The Velashape device precisely heats the underlying tissue within the targeted treatment area. This heat causes shrinkage and tightening of the fat cells and increased lymphatic drainage,

resulting in a reduction of the dimpled appearance of cellulite, smoothing of the skin's surface, and a reshaping and firming of the treated area.

The Velashape procedure takes around 40 minutes to 1 hour, with little or no downtime. Four to six initial Velashape treatments are performed at 1-week intervals. Maintenance procedures are then required at 6-month intervals.

Some patients report that the treatment feels like a warm deep-tissue massage. No anesthesia is required. The treated area may appear flushed or pink for a short while, and may feel warm for several hours after. Most Velashape patients can resume normal activities immediately.

## VELASMOOTH®

Velasmooth is a safe, FDA-approved non-invasive treatment for the reduction of cellulite and the smoothing of unwanted bumps and bulges. A Velasmooth treatment combines vacuum suction, mechanical rollers, and heating through infrared light and bipolar radio frequency (RF) energy.

Velasmooth is a cosmetic cellulite-reduction treatment that uses a machine with a handpiece that uses vacuum suction and massage from mechanical rollers to stimulate blood circulation in the treated area and reduce cellulite. This combined action increases the oxygen in the cells and massages the hypodermis (the deepest layer of the skin) to drain retained fluids through the body's lymphatic system. The heat from the infrared laser and the bipolar RF energy is directed under the skin, and

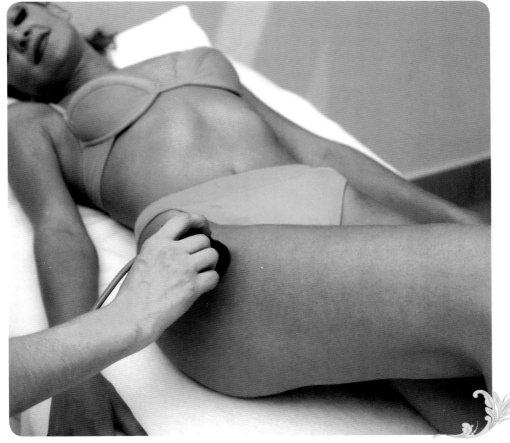

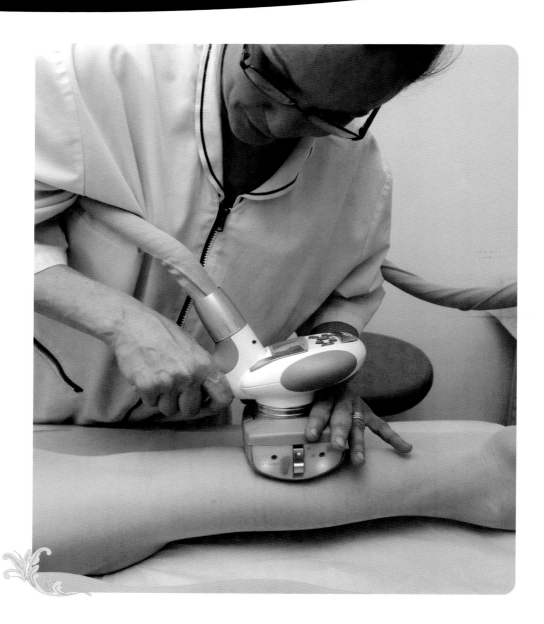

this releases energy stored in the fat calls, which results in the shrinkage of the cells, reducing the volume and the outward dimpled appearance of cellulite. After a few Velasmooth treatment sessions, the skin appears smoother, and the treated area is gradually reshaped and firmed.

Thighs, buttocks, calves, arms, and the abdomen can all benefit from Velasmooth cellulite-reduction treatment. Velasmooth is suitable for all skin types and skin colors.

The Velasmooth procedure reduces the appearance of cellulite and circumference of thighs, buttocks, arms, love handles, and the abdomen. Another effect of the Velasmooth procedure is improved circulation and relief from muscular aches and pains.

Up to 16 Velasmooth treatment sessions of between 45 and 60 minutes each are recommended initially, performed twice a week. The number of Velasmooth treatments required before individuals see results varies—some may not need the full 16 Velasmooth sessions to see improvements. Maintenance Velasmooth treatments are then usually performed once a month to achieve optimum results.

Some patients report that the Velasmooth cellulite reduction treatment feels like a warm deep-tissue massage. No anesthesia is required. The treated area may appear flushed or pink from the heat for a short while, and may feel warm for several hours after treatment. Most Velasmooth treatment patients can resume normal activities immediately.

## ENDERMOLOGIE®

French cosmetic surgeons developed the techniques used in Endermologie. The process is now patented in the U.S. as well. Endermologie uses rollers over problem areas of the skin. At the same time, suction is used to redistribute the skin and remove dimpling. Those opting for Endermologie usually need about 14 to 28 45-minute sessions to see results and must also have monthly treatments afterward.

## TRIACTIVE®

TriActive Laser Dermology incorporates three different methods for restoring a normal balance to the skin and outer layers, including smoothing and tightening. This triple-action treatment is designed to reduce the appearance of cellulite through the combined action of mechanical massage, localized cooling, and deep laser stimulation.

**The triple action includes:**

**Deep laser action**—the action of the six diode lasers enhances microcirculation.
**Mechanical massage**—the deep massaging and stimulating action on the subcutaneous tissue may result in a tighter appearance in the treated areas. This can be particularly noticeable when the treatments are done before and after liposuction procedures.
**Localized cooling**—cooling aids in smoothing the appearance of cellulite.

Smoothing and tightening can be accomplished in most areas of the body and face. These benefits are enhanced when combined with a healthy diet (including sufficient fluid intake) and exercise.

# BODY CONTOURING
## SmartLipo/Laser lipolysis

### WHY HAVE SMARTLIPO?

It is designed to treat localized fat using a cannula and laser technology which breaks down fat cells and reduces them to an oily substance that can be easily absorbed and expelled naturally by the patient's body.

## What is the procedure?

**SmartLipo fat treatment involves the use of a laser and cannula to dissolve localized pockets of fat and tighten the surrounding skin almost anywhere in the body.**

## SMARTLIPO/LASER LIPOLYSIS

As well as breaking down and expelling fat cells, the low-level laser energy used in SmartLipo also stimulates the production of new collagen. The result of SmartLipo treatment is a slimmer, more defined appearance.

The treatment is almost painless, and may be an alternative for people who wish to reduce their areas of fat without resorting to more invasive cosmetic surgery procedures such as conventional liposuction. As a result, the SmartLipo recovery time is minimal.

### SmartLipo treats localized pockets of fat in the:

- Face (except around the eyes)
- Chin
- Back of neck
- Upper arms
- Male breasts
- Tummy
- Waist
- Hips
- Buttocks
- Inner and outer thighs
- Pubic mound.

One to three SmartLipo treatment sessions are normally needed, with repeat sessions after a 3–6 month interval. SmartLipo differs from invasive surgical fat reduction procedures in that there is no general anesthesia required, there is minimal discomfort during the procedure, minimal post-procedure pain, minimal bleeding and bruising, no incisions or sutures are needed, and there is minimal recovery time, with most SmartLipo patients able to return to work within 24 hours.

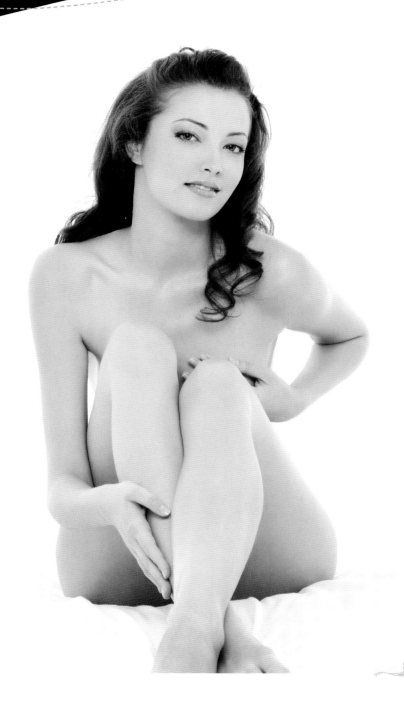

# FREQUENTLY ASKED QUESTIONS
*An overview*

**For answers to questions about anything from the history of cosmetic surgery to the costs involved, this section is the place to find general information on all things cosmetic surgery-related.**

### How can I minimize the effects of facial aging?

Nowhere does aging leave its imprint more noticeably than on the face. Sun exposure, as well as aging, contributes to facial wrinkling—as do certain lifestyle factors such as diet, the amount of alcohol you consume, and whether or not you smoke.

Facial rejuvenation surgery may involve procedures on the face and neck, eyelids, forehead, and eyebrow areas, as well as procedures to reduce fine lines on the skin. These procedures can often be performed at the same time as each other, or may be carried out in separate sessions.

The procedure, or combination of procedures, that is right for you will depend on your personal objectives and the opinion of your surgeon.

### Are looks really that important?

Most people would agree that what is on the inside of a person is more important than what is on the outside. But we are beginning to understand is that what is on the outside is quite important too, as it reflects the way we feel inside.

Cosmetic surgery is not about vain, self-indulgent narcissism. It's about ordinary people with problems—whether it's a nose that's too big, breasts that are too small, or wrinkled sagging skin that makes someone who feels young and alive look old and depressed. It could be a problem that you were born with, or one that comes with age. Cosmetic surgery can help ordinary people solve the problems with their appearance that make them unhappy; such surgical procedures can help you not only look better but feel better as well. They can often lead to improved self-esteem and increased self-confidence. Think of it as a little change on the outside that can lead to a big change on the inside. In summary, that is what cosmetic surgery is really all about: big changes... on the inside.

### Is cosmetic surgery for me?

Over the years, surgeons and psychologists have found that certain attitudes indicate that cosmetic surgery is appropriate for a patient.

Cosmetic surgery can improve your looks. It can help you look as young as you feel. And sometimes it can even boost your self-esteem and self-confidence. The rest is up to you. You should be realistic about what you'll look like afterward. Cosmetic surgery deals in improvement—not in perfection. If you can accept that, your surgery will be successful. If your expectations are realistic and you're doing it for the right reasons, the chances are excellent that you will be happy with your results.

## What causes wrinkles and sagging?

With age, various changes occur to the skin. Connective fibers located within the skin layers allow the skin to stretch and then return to its original shape. Over the years, these connective fibers decrease in number and they function less efficiently. The skin can no longer easily return to its former position after it is stretched. Time and age are the essential factors: a young person

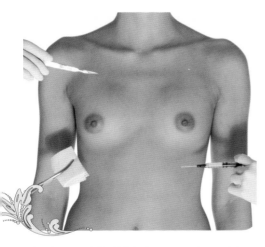

who loses 40 lb (20 kg) may end up with tight skin, while an older person, having lost the same amount of weight, will then be left with loose, hanging skin.

## What is a good age to have a facelift?

Most people requesting facelift surgery are between the ages of 45 and 60, although there are patients both younger and older

than that. About three-quarters of patients are women, although many more men have been turning to facelift surgery in recent times. Most patients are honest about their reasons for wanting facelift surgery. They hope that an operation to rejuvenate their appearance will make them look as young as they feel; they feel somehow that their facial appearance is betraying them.

Unrealistic expectations about the results of facial rejuvenation can only lead to disappointment. A complete consultation with a cosmetic surgeon will resolve the question of whether you are, potentially, a good candidate for a facelift.

## How will I know if a surgeon is right for me?

Having seen a number of surgeons, you should start to get a feeling about who is right for you. You should never forget that personal chemistry is very important in choosing your surgeon. Remember, your surgery will effectively be a journey, from the start of the operation to the end of recovery. You therefore need to feel reassured in the hands of any surgeon throughout the course of your journey. Choose one you feel comfortable with: someone who is easy to talk to; someone who is friendly yet professional; someone who listens closely to what you want and cares about what you need. The majority of cosmetic surgeons do. Do your homework and take your time, and you should have no problem finding an experienced, fully qualified and accredited surgeon who's right for you.

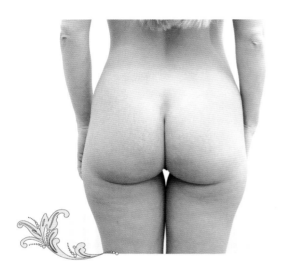

pain, although you may detect a light sensation of pressure at the site of the surgery. If sedation is administered as well (so-called "twilight anesthesia") then you will be asleep throughout most of the procedure and will not remember anything upon awakening.

Obviously if a general anesthetic is needed, then you will be completely asleep with the anesthetist monitoring you, and will not feel anything at all. After surgery, any pain you may experience can usually be controlled satisfactorily through medication and will gradually subside within a matter of days.

## I'm worried about looking unnatural or "plastic" after surgery. I don't want people to know. How can I be reassured?

Everybody has seen bad plastic surgery. You can spot it immediately... Instead of enhancing looks, the results almost certainly detract from them. Nobody wants to look as if they've obviously had cosmetic surgery. A good surgeon should be able to show you before and after pictures of past patients who display natural, well-balanced results, and not ones that leave a contrived or artificial look.

## Is cosmetic surgery painful?

During a local anesthetic procedure, the anesthetic that is administered ensures that you're comfortable and will feel no

## What happens if something goes wrong, or if I'm not happy with the results?

Complications can arise despite the best attempts of both doctor and patient to minimize these. No guarantees are given with any kind of surgery. However, if something were to go wrong, ensure that the cosmetic surgeon you have chosen can provide his or her surgical services to try to correct the problem. This should be a service offered at no extra expense to you. Similarly, if after all the factors of healing and settling have taken place, the final result is not what you and your surgeon hoped for, and providing that there is room for surgical maneuver to improve the result, your surgeon should offer to rectify this at no cost to you. However, anesthesiology fees, surgery center charges, implants, and any other ancillary expenses may remain the responsibility of the patient.

**Is cosmetic surgery covered by insurance?**
When a cosmetic surgery procedure is being performed for cosmetic reasons, insurance will not cover this. If the surgery is necessary for reconstructive purposes, it may be partially or fully covered by insurance (individual insurance policies vary; do check with your insurer). Cosmetic surgery procedures that may be covered by insurance include breast reconstruction (after a mastectomy), rhinoplasty (for breathing problems), tummy tuck surgery (for gastric bypass patients), and eyelid surgery (to correct vision problems).

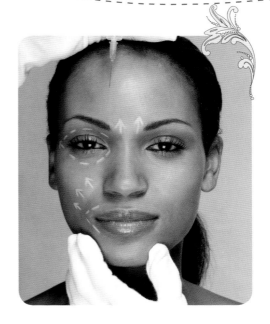

**Where should cosmetic surgery be performed?**
That can depend on the surgeon. Most cosmetic surgeons are affiliated with local hospitals and can arrange operating room times as needed. Many have similar arrangements at surgical centers, while other surgeons have private surgery suites in their own office spaces. You will find that many cosmetic surgeons fit into all or most of these categories, and offer options tailored to each patient. They will help you choose your surgery location based on comfort, safety, scheduling issues, or geographical concerns.

**Is cosmetic surgery performed on an "outpatient" or "inpatient" basis?**
Most cosmetic surgery procedures are performed on an outpatient basis. In some cases, usually when the surgery is

very extensive or complications arise, an overnight stay might be required.

**Is there a "right" age to pursue cosmetic surgery?**
There is no age rule involved when it comes to wanting to have cosmetic surgery. Each procedure should be determined on a case-by-case basis, looking at the individual's unique body type and response to the aging process. Of course, there are age tendencies for certain procedures. Facelifts generally are not performed on patients under 30—mini-lifts or laser procedures might be suggested instead—but this is not a hard and fast rule. Otoplasty (ear surgery), on the other hand, is appropriate for adults or patients as young as five years old. Cosmetic surgery is very much an individual choice, based on individual circumstances.

# RESOURCES & INDEX

## UNITED STATES

**American Society for Aesthetic Plastic Surgery:**
www.surgery.org

**American Society of Plastic Surgeons:**
www.plasticsurgery.org

**American Academy of Dermatology:**
www.aad.org

**American Academy of Facial Plastic and Reconstructive Surgery:**
www.aafprs.org

**American Society for Dermatological Surgery:**
www.asds.net

## UNITED KINGDOM

**The British Association of Aesthetic Plastic Surgeons (BAAPS):**
www.baaps.org

**The British Association of Plastic, Reconstructive and Aesthetic Plastic Surgeons:**
www.bapras.org.uk

**The Royal College of Surgeons of England:**
www.rcseng.ac.uk

**Medicine and Healthcare Products Regulatory Agency:**
www.siliconereview.gov.uk

**Department of Health:**
www.dh.gov.uk

**Healthcare Commission:**
www.healthcarecommission.org.uk

**The General Medical Council:**
www.gmc-uk.org

**British Association of Cosmetic Doctors:**
www.cosmeticdoctors.co.uk

**British Association of Dermatologists:**
www.bad.org.uk

**British Association of Oral and Maxillofacial Surgeons:**
www.baoms.org.uk

## INTERNATIONAL

**The International Association of Aesthetic Plastic Surgeons:**
www.isaps.org

**International Confederation of Plastic, Reconstructive and Aesthetic Surgery:**
http://www.ipras.org/

**The European Association of Plastic Surgeons:**
www.euraps.org

**European Society of Plastic, Reconstructive and Aesthetic Surgeons:**
http://www.espras.org/

## OTHER

**Professor James Frame— Plastic and Reconstructive Surgeon:**
www.professorjamesframe.co.uk

**Dr. Edgardo Schiavone— Plastic Surgeon:**
www.edgardoschiavone.com

**Dr. Bessam Farjo—Hair Transplant Surgeon:**
www.farjo.net

**An aesthetic service group:**
www.skindeep.me.uk

**A beauty website:**
www.ambeautysite.com

**Medical device groups:**
http://www.q-med.com/
http://www.radiesse.com/
http://www.teoxane.com/
www.merzpharma.co.uk

**A pharmaceutical company:**
http://www.allergan.co.uk/

**Medical device products:**
http://www.velashape.com/
http://www.velasmooth.com/
www.cosmoderm.co.za
http://www.elevess.com/
http://www.mentorcorp.com/
www.sculptra.co.uk
www.endermologie.com
www.cynosure.com
www.thermage.com

# INDEX & CREDITS

## Quintet would like to acknowledge the following:

Shutterstock 1-5; Shutterstock 8; Shutterstock 11; Mehau Kulyk/Science Photo Library 12; Unattributed engraving/Mary Evans Picture Library 13; The Sketch, 1907, all image/Illustrated London News Ltd/Mary Evans Picture Library 14; Skin graft operation, from 'Selecta Praxis Medico-Chirurgica' by Alexander Auvert, Paris, 1856 (coloured engraving), French School, (19th century)/Bibliotheque de la Faculte de Medecine, Paris, France/London News Ltd/Mary Evans 15; Mark Thomas/Science Photo Library 17; Cristina Pedrazzini/Science Photo Library 18; Adam Gault/SPL 21; Shutterstock 24; Mark Fairey/Alamy 27; Stockbyte 28; Science Photo Library/Alamy 31; image100/Alamy 32; Duane Reader/Getty Images 33; Floresco Productions/Getty Images 35; Shutterstock 36; Professor James Frame 37; Professor James Frame 38; Professor James Frame 39; Christian Weigel/Corbis 40; Shutterstock 42; Shutterstock 51; Shutterstock 57; Shutterstock 65; Shutterstock 69; Q-Med 71; Adam Gault/SPL 72; Shutterstock 79; Shutterstock 85; Shutterstock 87; Dr. Edgardo Schiavone 94; Shutterstock 96; Science Photo Library 98; Adam Gault/SPL 101; Dr. Edgardo Schiavone 105; Dr. Edgardo Schiavone 108; Paul Viant/Getty Images 109; Dennis Guyitt/istockphoto.com 119; Shutterstock 126; Shutterstock 128; Corbis RF/Alamy 131; image100/Alamy 135; Dr. Edgardo Schiavone 138; Pascal Goetgheluck/Science Photo Library 143; Shutterstock 151; Dr. Edgardo Schiavone 156; Science Photo Library/Alamy 159; Shutterstock 168; STOCK4B GmbH/Alamy 173; Louise Gubb/Corbis 176; Barron Claiborne/Corbis 181; Shutterstock 182; Sean Justice/Corbis 184; Lea Suzuki/San Francisco Chronicle/Corbis 186; Professor James Frame 187; Science Photo Library/Alamy 188; www.farjo.net 196; Medical-on-Line/Alamy 199; John Millard MD 200; Louis Quail/Corbis 202; Dr. Edgardo Schiavone 204; Professor James Frame 206; Science Photo Library/Alamy 207; Science Photo Library/Alamy 208; Amelie Benoist/Science Photo Library, Amelie Benoist/Science Photo Library 211; Shutterstock 212; Shutterstock 214; Shutterstock 218; Shutterstock 222; Adam Gault/SPL 224; AJ Photo/Hop Americain/Science Photo Library 227; Milk Photographie/Corbis 229; aStra productions /Corbis 230; Image Source/Jupiterimages 235; aStra productions/Corbis 237; BSIP, Laurent/Laeticia/Science Photo Library 238; imagebroker/Alamy 241; Stock Connection Blue/Alamy 243; Mendil/Science Photo Library 244; Shutterstock 247

All other images are the copyright of Quintet Publishing plc. While every effort has been made to credit contributors, Quintet would like to apologize should there be any omissions or errors, and would be pleased to make the appropriate correction for future editions of the book.

I wish to thank the all of the organizations, medical professionals, and individuals who have kindly collaborated with me in providing information and research for the Cosmetic Surgery Companion, namely: Professor James Frame—Plastic and Reconstructive Surgeon, and Dr. Marco La Malfa, Consultant Anesthetist and Cosmetic Doctor, with thanks also to Dr. Edgardo Schiavone, John Millard MD, Stephen Goldstein MD, Dr Farjo Bessam, Farjo Medical Centre, The Private Clinic London, ISAPS, BAAPS, BAPRAS, BACD, and The Lavenham Clinic and Spa—Suffolk. With special thanks to Marco, Alessio, and Jasmine La Malfa for inspiring me every day.

Antonia Mariconda